Life Rolls On

Life Rolls On

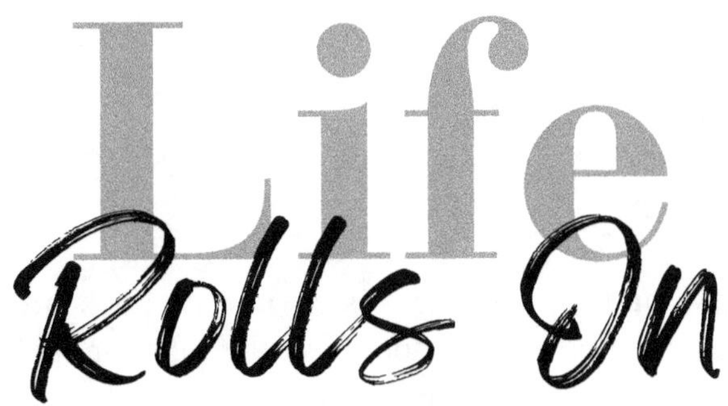

Richard P. Mason
and
Briana Mason

gatekeeper press™

Columbus, Ohio

Life Rolls On

Published by Gatekeeper Press
2167 Stringtown Rd, Suite 109
Columbus, OH 43123-2989
www.GatekeeperPress.com

Library of Congress Control Number:2022931755

ISBN (paperback): 9781662925481
eISBN: 9781662925498

DEDICATION

To the woman who made all the dreams shared on these pages not only possible, but a reality – my wife, Nancy.

You are the best thing that I lucked into; a true life partner, a nurturing mother, a patient caregiver and assistant.

I suspect that you represent a large group of unsung heroes, and I love you for all that you are.

Contents

PROLOGUE

The intent of this book is threefold.

The first: to provide examples to disabled folks, whether maverick or veteran, of what is still possible; that there are still plenty of new adventures and beautiful upsides to experience.

Next: to educate the general public of the capabilities physically challenged individuals possess, even and especially after having experienced a life-altering accident.

The last: simply to entertain, and share my story with those who are willing to listen.

All of the chapters and stories within actually occurred, and only some are slightly embellished for understanding and effect.

I encourage all who read these pages to attempt to put themselves in the place of the author, to gain a glimpse into the lives of those affected by an SCI. Individuals experiencing such an event do not want to be given special treatment, but to be further understood and be considered a valued part of society. Their goal is to contribute to the overall betterment of their community and ecosphere.

CHAPTER 1

THE TRANSITION

It was a warm early summer evening at the beginning of June, in Erie, Pennsylvania, 1976. I was cruising on my Kawasaki 175 motorcycle, heading to my shift at Firch's Bakery, thinking ahead to a long, hot night of making bread from scratch. Even though the sun would be fast asleep, I knew it would still be muggy and miserable for the duration. The summer was shaping up to be exactly like the evening shift that lay ahead. Not mild, to put it mildly. It was only week two.

In order to pay for college, my summer job between freshman and sophomore year, I was working at Firch's. I was on the swing shift, from 11pm through 7am. My task was simple: make fresh buns for McDonald's, Burger King and other restaurants. Specifically, I was to take 5-pound baking trays, capable of holding 24 balls of dough each, arranged in 6 rows of 4. I would then load them onto a conveyor belt in quick succession, while the "Chopper" rhythmically dropped seeming-perfectly round balls into each cup on the tray.

The machine got the name the "Chopper", among the employees, because of the stainless steel "gate" that was responsible for systematically dropping the dough. It ensured that only one row, four dough balls, was dropped at a time. Imagine a tollbooth arm, on a dough ball conveyor belt. However, occasionally at the end of an individual run the machine would lose the flour used to keep the balls of dough from sticking. This meant, another of the tray loaders' other responsibilities was to reach in between chops to un-jam the dough without stopping the belt or losing digits by moving too slowly. I was informed that the bakery had an insurance policy in place. This seemingly over-the-top policy was in case the dreaded happened; the tray loader didn't retract his fingers in time when unsticking the dough from the machine. From the tip of the finger to the first knuckle was worth $3000, the second knuckle $6000, and the entire finger was worth $15,000, according to one rumor. But no one could confirm or deny the exact dollar amount. Part of the folklore was about "Willie", a tray loader that needed a new car. As the story goes, he decided that his pinky finger was worth a new ride. No, my nickname wasn't Willie, but Willie and I have also never been seen in the same room together.

That particular night at work was tedious and uneventful. Little did I know what the hours following would have in store for me. As my shift was ending, and I was relieved of duty, I opened the bakery door to a refreshing early morning breeze and the sounds of birds waking to a new day. It was blissful. I decided to stop by McDonalds to sample one of the buns I had helped to create the night before. I mounted my bike, which was the cheapest way to get from point A to point B while having a little fun. After a speedy breakfast, it was shaping up to be a beautiful 75° day, especially for early summer. The perfect day to head to the beach at Presque Isle, on Lake Erie. As a result, I decided to cruise by my good buddy Mike's house to check in and see if he was up for some fun in the sun. As it turns out, he was more than interested in the idea. We made plans to head out to Presque Isle that afternoon and splash around at the beach together. I headed towards home to grab a quick nap, lunch and change of clothes before heading out for the rest of the day. Along the way, I cruised past a different friend's house, in the neighborhood, and saw him in the front yard doing his chores for the day. He explained that they had just filled their four foot above ground "doughboy" pool. I suspect he would have done pretty much anything to get out of those chores, but this worked out better for all involved. The water was fresh, and he suggested that we should stay there to swim, instead of making the 26-mile trek, round trip, to the beach. It sounded like a good idea at the time, and much less work, so a group of four guys decided to keep it local.

We reconvened in the early afternoon, around the doughboy, and started acting like testosterone filled 18-year-olds tend to, when in packs. We were running up to the side of the pool, planting our feet, springing up and over the side and diving in without touching the sides. It was my turn, and I ran up and brazenly sprung over the side of the pool, gliding sleekly along the bottom, and back up to the top. I thought I looked pretty suave. The others, who were sitting on the side of the pool, disagreed. They all started taunting, questioning, "is that the best you can do"? And, of course, being 18 years old, full of testosterone, and competitive whether it came to sports or just laundry, I was up to the challenge of going bigger and better … or so I thought.

On my next attempt, I ran a little harder, jumped a little higher, planning to curl around past the bottom similar to the 1st attempt. However, simple physics would tell you that the added height and speed made for a faster than anticipated entry into the water, not allowing enough time to curl around, and safely clear the bottom.

I felt the sudden, excruciatingly painful clunk, my body shivered and went completely numb, as my head squarely hit the bottom.

At that moment, my life would be forever changed, paradoxically in dramatic yet anticlimactic fashion.

Immediately realizing there was a monumental problem, as I attempted to stand, and grab the side of the pool, I realized I was unable to do so, with severely weakened arms. My formerly athletic legs, and general build would no longer support me. Could no longer support me. They simply hung limp below me. I was confused, to say the least. As I feebly tried to tread water and yell for any and all help, I realized that my friends thought I was pranking. What else do 18 year old friends do on summer break? Of course they thought it was a poorly executed joke. After a few minutes, what little strength I had in my arms had given out, and I was no longer going to be able to keep my head above water. My hope of help was sinking with me. I struggled for each breath of air, knowing that I would soon be completely submerged. Still thinking I was kidding, my friends started laughing and splashing at me. To state the obvious, they weren't taking the garbled cries for help into serious consideration. They promptly pulled their feet out of the pool, stood up and headed to the garage. They were going to check out a newly restored MBGGT. In my mind I said final goodbyes to anyone and everyone I could think of in those desperate moments, and that I would see them on the other side. I promptly passed out and slowly floated to rest on the bottom of the pool. I quickly lost consciousness. After 3 or 4 minutes they realized that no one, not even I, could hold their breath that long and quickly pulled me out of the pool. It would be at a later point in time that a doctor would tell me that more damage had likely been done to my spinal cord in their haste to get me out of the water. However you slice it, I was pulled out of the water in time to spare my life.

To stabilize my severely broken neck, in the ambulance they placed sandbags on either side of my head. Not exactly the most medically sound practice by today's standards, and they weren't quite tight enough. My head rocked back and forth with each bump we came across in the road, and it was enough to make me stir and waken at one point. The medics tightened the bags and I promptly passed out again. The next time I regained consciousness I was in the ICU. I was surrounded by medical personnel, with lights flashing, beeping machines and buzzers, I started to realize the true seriousness of the situation. Suddenly, I heard a drill starting up. I thought to myself, "What the hell? They could at least wait until I'm out of the room before they do remodeling and repairs". And it was at just that moment, I felt the drill start to grind into my skull. It needs to be said that I was none too keen on the sounds, the intense sensation, or the knowledge that I was having lifechanging work done to my body. They had been waiting for me to wake up to ensure that, in case they drilled a little bit too deep, they didn't pith my brain like a frog in sophomore biology. You can imagine what was going through my mind. They were putting in traction tongs designed to stabilize my neck, when I again promptly passed out.

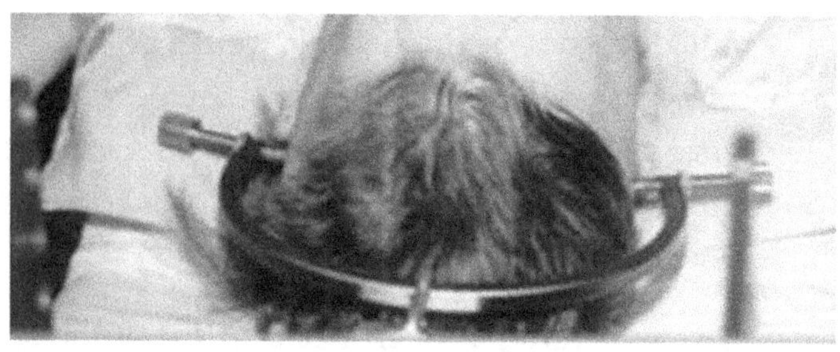

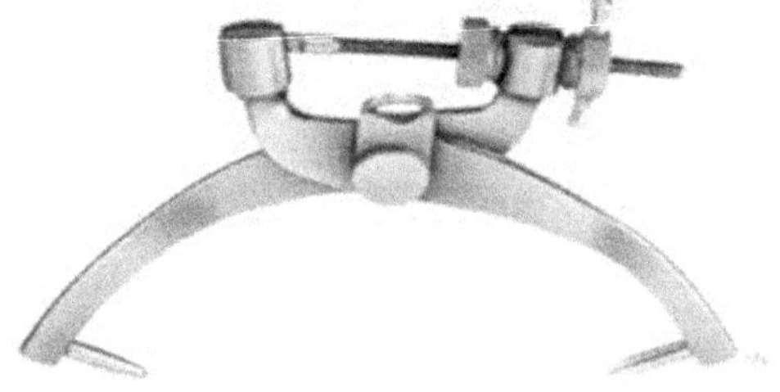

The ultimate result of the accident was that I was now completely paralyzed from the chest down; unable to stand, walk or independently move my legs and, with limited function in my weakened hands and arms. In other words, my brain could no longer successfully, and directly, communicate with my appendages, for the most part.

The entirety of my activity of the next six weeks included me laying strictly flat on top of a cot-like frame, which measured the length of my body. This is where the newly placed traction atop my head came into play; it was connected to a rope, which was stretched over a pulley wheel and made a 90° turn towards the floor. At the bottom of the rope were home gym-like weights, and their purpose was to provide traction. Every two hours, like clockwork, the hospital staff would come into the room, attach a second similarly-sized cot to the top, strap me into the contraption, and then flip me over, like a pancake being flipped in a skillet. The traction and flipping were performed with the intent of preventing bed sores and were continued militantly throughout the days for the duration of the six weeks.

The only reason it continued for as long as it did, the full six weeks, is because someone on staff had misread an x-ray. Due to this mistake, they were waiting for the C-6/7 spinal process bone to heal and stabilize my neck. The bone they were waiting for had unfortunately had been completely severed on impact and could not re-fuse. Subsequent x-rays that followed finally allowed a clear review and diagnosis. Somebody, although I'm not sure who, realized the bone they were waiting to re-fuse wasn't there anymore. At that point, the only option was to head off to surgery to put in a metal rod to stabilize the neck.

After the surgery site had healed, then began the long, grueling process of rehabilitation therapy. Each day began with the ritual of relearning how to get dressed. This took upwards of 2 hours, because I could no longer use my arms, legs and fingers, and had to lay flat in bed. I was unable to sit up, at least for the time being. I wasn't yet strong enough. As an example, putting on 1 single sock could take 30 minutes, and that was on a good day. Take a brief moment to think about how many things you get done in 30 minutes during your morning routine. I was now never going to speed through any of these mundane tasks again.

These items, along with other non-essential articles of clothing, quickly became superfluous. Putting on a pair of pants suddenly became an adventure, on a daily basis. It required lying in bed and placing the pants over my feet and inching them up my legs while rolling side to side. This was not quick, nor was it glamorous. Shoe preference changed from my favorite Chuck Taylor All Stars to slippers, simply for ease of adornment. As the decades passed, my chronically swollen feet kept slippers a front runner for daily footwear. The process of dressing quickly shifted from form to function.

After getting dressed, sometimes well into the afternoon, it was off to physical therapy, on a gurney, where I was placed each time on a "tilt table". This device was designed to reintroduce verticality into my life. After six weeks of lying flat, you can't just sit up straight immediately. A tilt of as little as 15° from horizontal would cause the room to be set in motion, and I could lose consciousness. It took me an entire week to work up to a sitting position. Then it was time for the real work to begin. Physical therapy sessions lasted two hours at a time, if not longer. There were many baby steps along the way. For example one activity and goal was getting from lying flat and working my way to a sitting position. This started with me laying flat on a mat, on my back, and learning how to rhythmically swing my arms back and forth, rolling side to side, eventually gaining enough momentum to get over to my side. That was the midway point of the exercise. From that point, I had to grab my legs behind the knees and pull them tight to my chest, and then work my way to a sitting position. After painstaking effort, and more than a little bit of failure, it was only one short week until I reached my goal, and successfully, semi-efficiently got myself into a sitting position.

After gaining the ability to sit up the next step was to be able to transfer over to a wheelchair and on to the weight machines to, at least minimally, rebuild my weakened arms. You can imagine that if going from lying flat to sitting upright took one week, that these other activities took a significant amount of time to "master".

One hour of each day was dedicated to Occupational Therapy, which was different from rehabilitation and physical therapies that I participated in. This involved relearning how to successfully complete ADL's, or activities of daily living, such as learning how to hold a pen, brush my teeth, and maximizing use out of my fingers. My fine motor was all but eliminated, and it was important to recapture what I could. It's amazing how easy it is to take little things for granted before you no longer have them at your disposal. At the start of the process, it would take close to an hour just to complete what I chose to incorporate into my morning routine. The other function of OT was to evaluate the remaining physical skills I had and determine how to break them down and re-assimilate them with other basic skills like eating, bathing, and toileting. I affectionately called it learning how to put round pegs in square holes. In what seemed like an impossibility, as I struggled to write my name, we started conversations about potential occupations that were feasible with my levels of function and capabilities.

As you can probably imagine, this newfound situation was less than ideal. One of the main things that made it somewhat bearable was the support of my family and true friends. My mother was my biggest supporter and advocate. She would come every day after she got off work, rain or shine, just to sit and be with her youngest child. It meant more to me than I could express at the time. The concern for me was evident on her face, even though she did her best to hide it. Conversely, there was an interesting turnover of friends after the accident. Some distanced themselves because, for various reasons, they just couldn't handle the "new me", or others that weren't as close of friends as I previously thought. I had held some of my friends in too high regard, but I would try my hardest not to repeat history in the interpersonal arena. In an odd way, this allowed me to reflect on my relationships with others and generally how I approached them, and how I should change that approach going forward. I gained much needed perspective. I was on my way to earning my engineering degree, fairly good at sports, and could usually find a date on Saturday night without too much effort. I admit that I looked at others for what they could do for me, as opposed to who they were and the series of life events made them that way, and potentially how we could be mutually beneficial to each other. After the accident, and really throughout my life, others stepped in and offered assistance where and how they could. There was only so much others could do at that point, as there was a lot I had to work through on my own, both physically and mentally. Even so, I did appreciate all of the help that was offered and given. I made friends with hospital orderlies, Tom and Pin, who would come by and help fill the quiet lonely nights and risk losing their job to bring late-night pizzas, margaritas and daiquiris. It seemed as though the adage make new friends but keep the old was at least partially true. My new life was bringing in new people that I both wanted and needed.

I remember in particular, one Saturday afternoon shortly after I began rehabbing, a group of friends stopped by to kidnap me from the hospital and go to the park across the street to get some fresh air. They just happened to have brought a cooler with cold beer and funny smelling cigarettes along with them. We spent the afternoon imbibing, listening to one of them play a guitar, not particularly well I might add, and enjoying a beautiful summer day. The park was situated in somewhat of a bowl, nestled at the bottom of a small hill. When it was time to go back, no one was quite sure how to get up the inclined sidewalk and out of the park, while successfully maneuvering an occupied wheelchair. Not knowing any better, I suggested getting a running start and use the momentum to get up the path. So, with a running start we headed up sidewalk and about halfway out the front wheels started wobbling and fluttering. They almost immediately turned sideways and then locked up, sending me flying through the air. The beer that I had been drinking prior, situated between my legs, landed on the incline above me. I watched as it slowly started trickling back down the hill toward me and I knew me getting soaked was inevitable. I had picked a bad day to wear white overalls. A mixture of blood and beer quickly covered me. This, along with the fact that I was wearing a soft collar neck brace to stabilize the newly repaired neck, was cause for concern about further damage, as it wasn't sturdy when it came to a booze-induced collision. They quickly scrambled to get me back in the chair and return to the hospital, crossing all fingers that it was without incurring even more injury. When the doors opened to the elevator on the rehab floor, I got off and all eyes in the waiting room turned towards me, aghast with the most alarmed looks on their faces. I explained to the nurses that I had "accidentally" fallen out of my chair. But as I was recounting the story it quickly became apparent that they weren't buying the story and the subject was dropped, never to be discussed again.

Since the incident occurred early in June, and the rehabilitation process was prolonged for several obvious reasons, I spent the bicentennial Fourth of July, 1976, in addition to my 19th birthday in the hospital, staring out the window. My thoughts were mostly on how life would really look once I emerged from the nest that rehab had become.

One day I was lying in bed and a stranger entered my room and introduced himself as Art. It became apparent from the civilian clothes that he was not affiliated with the hospital, but my interest had been piqued. We talked for awhile and he told me that he was a painter by trade and captained ships from Lake Erie to Florida for the wealthy. He inquired about my interests and whether I enjoyed swimming, and then further prodded if I'd like to try it when I was discharged. There was an immediate flashback to my most recent swimming experience, and the feeling of my face and head sinking below the water line as I descended to the bottom of the pool. I rudely said, "hey, I just got done fucking drowning, don't think so". He turned to me and calmly stated, "oh, you're not ready" and then quietly walked out the door. I barked at him for an explanation, but none was forthcoming.

The rehab process was incremental in nature and the relatively rapid progress at the beginning started to slow. About two months into my stay, during a "team" meeting I inquired about how much longer to expect. I was not ready for the response from the doctor. "Well individuals with your type of injury (C6/7 quadriplegia) have an average length of stay of 1 to 1 ½ years". WHAT? My mind was spinning; crunching numbers and everything else that I had lost, or was facing losing. "There's no way I'm staying here for another year", I blurted out. He replied, "Sorry, that's the process". But no further detail. It was at that point I made a commitment to prove him wrong. In short time, I became nothing short of a belligerent patient, questioning everything and sometimes outright refusing orders or instructions. Not to mention the trips out with friends, which heavily increased in frequency. After a couple months of battling and misbehavior, we came to a mutual understanding, it was time for me to be discharged. The 1 year estimate had shrunk significantly; to almost exactly four months. I had learned the basics and felt that the rest could be learned on the street, by trial and error. Or trial by fire.

I left rehab relying on a bag strapped to my leg to collect urine, the other end of the toileting experience was being handled through suppositories. Neither of which I could do independently. I was turned over to the custody of my parents. They were now in the position of helping their adult child with toileting needs, among the laundry list of other items.

CHAPTER 2

COLLEGE DAZE

It was a quiet Sunday morning well into winter, and outside was one of those snowstorms that you get used to growing up in an area like those that surround the Great Lakes. Those of you who are from the West Coast or the South, you would never survive. Big, bold and beautiful snowflakes gently floating to the ground, blanketing the landscape. It really is a beautiful, unique sight to behold. The only problem was the sheer volume of snow in each successive flurry. The ever-increasing frequency and persistence complicated the fact that I was scheduled to leave that afternoon to resume college.

"There's no way they're going to have school tomorrow", was the phrase my father voiced on a continuous loop. Throughout the morning, he would gaze out the window, loyally monitoring the weather. I replied to him, "Dad, this is really important to me". Looking at it as an opportunity to somewhat rejoin mainstream society, I was counting on this. I looked forward to resuming a "normal schedule" and days filled with something other than various forms of therapy. This was going to be my first time living away from home, let alone with a newfound disability. Not knowing what to expect in this future chapter, I felt it even more important to follow their schedule to a T. Finally worn down, he reluctantly agreed. He was more nervous than he let on, a palpable reluctance radiated off of him. I resumed putting the finishing touches on my luggage and before we knew it the car was crammed full, and we were heading down I-90 toward Edinboro University and the restart of life. No big deal. The campus was only 20 miles away from home. Meaning it was a minimal springing from the nest, but nonetheless vital to me. My mental well-being was tied to this rite of passage. But the continually accumulating snow and increasing winds were presenting a major challenge. The front bumper of the car had begun pushing powder, transforming before our very eyes into a snowplow. We slowly inched down the freeway. As the minutes ticked away, it seemed like we would never arrive.

We eventually found the campus, and my future home, nestled in Shafer Hall. The only evidence of the adjoining parking lot, were the heaps of snow that covered what we all assumed were cars, looking like a miniature white mountain range. The closest we could get to the front door of the dorm was 100 feet away in what seemed like the last parking spot in the state of Pennsylvania. The sidewalk leading up to the dormitory entrance was covered with three feet of snow, easily. The only sign of life: a narrow track in the middle that had been trampled by people scurrying in and out. This left a paltry path about half the width of my chair. With my father in back, pushing, and my mother in front, pulling, as a team we inched our way toward the entrance. It was a repeat performance of our drive over.

The feeling of victory was small but well earned, as we pushed the button for the motorized front doors, and they swung open, sweeping the accumulated snow aside.

Just inside the door sat an older gentleman with salt-and-pepper hair and beard. His body violently jerked appearing as though his arms and legs were dancing on strings, like a marionette. Prior to this, the only people that I had known in wheelchairs were old people who were no longer able to walk. Feeling uncomfortable I purposefully tried to avoid eye contact as he attempted to communicate with severely garbled speech. Was this going to be how people viewed our interactions?

We continued down a narrow hallway and up a short ramp to two doors that led to the dormitory rooms, finally. The two doors opened to the common rooms where people gathered, comparing notes about events that had transpired over the holiday break and about their classes scheduled for the upcoming semester.

The extent of my worldly belongings, which had filled the car to the brim, sat in the corner dwarfed by the empty dorm room. As our conversation reverberated off the wall, I tried to put on a brave face as my parents looked back over their shoulders at me with obvious concern. Simultaneously, they opened the door to leave, wanting to avoid the ever-worsening weather, but obviously conflicted. As the door shut behind them, I sat alone in the middle of the empty, unadorned room with each sound seemingly multiplying the size of the room as it bounced off the blank walls, wondering what I had gotten myself into.

Suddenly, I was brought back to the present by an abrupt knock on the door. As I opened the door, the person who stood there identified himself as Buck, and invited me to join a small gathering of students. To be clear, it was NOT a party. We headed down the hallway together and knocked at the door, with loud voices behind it that were hard to ignore. The door eventually opened wide, and we were welcomed in by unidentified voices and a waft of smoke. Surveying the room, I noticed 4 overwhemingly average looking individuals in chairs, gathered around the bed in the middle of the room. On the desk in the corner there was a case of beer next to a window, with a string attached to it. On the other end of the string hung a cloth bag full of beers, outside the window, chilling in nature's refrigerator. How innovative. Someone threw a baggie of buds on the bed and the adjustment to the new normal had begun, just like that. It seemed almost as smooth as the snow that continued to pile up outside.

The snowstorm continued throughout that night, and we awoke the next day to four feet of snow piled up to the window ledge. We were effectively snowed in for the next week. What a welcome to college life. Apparently, it was more time to adjust to the social aspect of school, not necessarily the academia.

Looking out from the dorm room windows, you could see the university cafeteria which was directly across the street. Since none of us were able to leave the building, they fed us by bringing the cafeteria offering of the day, packaged in portioned Styrofoam containers. By the time the food reached the dorm the initially unappealing culinary offerings were always cold, since they were out in the elements. But we managed to survive as long as we had an a.b. (short for able-bodied) individual willing to forge out into the waist-deep winter-land to restock the beer supply, and the phones were working for the daily pizza delivery. We opted for the cheesy delicacy after receiving each frosty plate of mystery food. Piles of unopened cafeteria food containers, empty pizza boxes and empty beer bottles began to line and litter the hallway, faster than the snow was falling outside.

After a week of seclusion amongst all of our dormmates, the snow had finally been re-piled and we were eventually able to make our initial venture outside, and into a more traditional college life. One day, I noticed an individual, later to be identified as Steve, my future neighbor. One day I happened to notice him directing and coordinating the movement of two large boxes. Shortly thereafter, the music began. Once it started it didn't stop, lasting for two entire semesters at one volume: loud. His stereo also had a turntable that played his entire collection, three whole LPs, on repeat. Since we heard them over and over, again and again, we memorized those LPs quickly.

All of this was happening back in the day before the ADA (Americans with Disabilities Act) was enacted. Every state had its own way of addressing the "issue" and burden of affording accessibility. Edinboro University was one of two identified campuses dedicated to accessibility in Pennsylvania. The state's attempt to make college life accessible was to fully adapt one campus on each side of the state with automatic doors, ramps into buildings, curb cuts placed sporadically around campus to provide access to the sidewalks and support personnel known as "floaters" designated to assist students with physical challenges. We were transported to classes in the back of ramped vans. The University also offered academic support, including notetakers and additional test taking time, if necessary. Those students requiring assistance with activities of daily living (A.D.L.'s) were contacted by, and set up with, appropriate resources and a floater. Each dorm room was equipped with a buzzer system which was connected to a central location and used to summon help in the event that we needed it without prior notification. New students were required to live in the dorms for their first two years in school. Even with the accommodations making life and the transition a little more bearable, everyone looked forward to the day that they could make the move off campus.

A favorite learning tool was affectionately called "Study with a Buddy", and it was held at The Hotel. The Hotel was a local bar that offered $1 pitchers during happy hour. An unheard of deal with today's rate. People showed up with the intention of studying. But after the first pitcher, the books slowly disappeared from the table and the "studying" effectively was converted into a night of partying. This became a routine occurrence. One academic principle was proven over and over during these happy hour study sessions; there's a direct positive correlation between late night parties and the number of early morning classes missed the next day. I somehow managed to not only survive, but pass enough classes to be awarded a diploma.

My first job after graduation was working at a social services agency in downtown Erie. Although located only 15 miles away, that drive could turn into a 1hr+ adventure with the arrival of an unexpected snowstorm The trip usually only took between 20 and 30 minutes on an average day. On Christmas Eve after finishing a half day at work, I decided to stop by my brother's house for some innocent holiday cheer, only to find that he had been called into work. After I struck out at Tom's, I stopped by the homes of other family that lived in town, all without success. It had begun to snow, creating a wintry holiday wonderland. But even though the snow looked so beautiful, it never truly made for a clean fairytale. So, I decided to take the backroads through the countryside on my way back home. All the while, I was sampling one of the beers situated in the backseat. With holiday jingles on the radio, I sledded down the road. As my front bumper began to push snow, I realized that if I got stuck it might be a while before anybody came along to the rescue, so I decided it was time to head home. Pulling into the parking lot that was mostly empty since students were home for the holidays, I parked in a prime spot right next to the entrance. The snow was so deep by this point that I was unable to fully open my driver side door, and barely managed to squeeze my folding wheelchair out the door. Unable to roll through the piled up snow I was forced to get out of my chair and crawl, my wheelchair in tow behind me. To add to the degree of difficulty I had lost my gloves and was barehanded. I woke the next morning with a bit of frostbite on my hand. The snow had proven once again that it was beautiful yet menacing. I had known some who had even more intense stories of battling the beautiful white flakes. Since these instances happened all too frequently, thoughts of sunny California danced in the back of my mind. I was keen on avoiding the wrath of nature as much as possible. But with my mom's declining health and recent negative prognosis, I just couldn't see being on the other side of the country. I was hopeful that somehow my mom's health would improve, and that I would be able to make my way to the west coast without hesitation. My mom was the one who helped me after my accident, and throughout my entire life. I was her baby, and I wanted her to forever be there, even though we all knew that was an impossibility, the ultimate impracticality of life. Even with all of this at the forefront, California continued to call, loudly.

CHAPTER 3

WESTWARD HO

It was fall of 1981, and my mother had finally succumbed to her illness about half a year prior. I had taken some time to mourn her passing and sort out my life, where I truly wanted to go from there. The loss of a parent forces you to face your mortality, all the while simultaneously wanting to do big things. Better things. Maybe it is a way to honor what your loved one did in this life and tell them that you won't waste what they accomplished; that it helped pave your way and is a steppingstone in your path to these amazing things. I sat down at the kitchen table one Sunday morning with my father and informed him of my intentions. "Dad I'm thinking about moving to California", I blatantly stated. I expanded on what I had shared, by saying that being in a chair naturally pairs with certain physical obstacles like stairs, curbs, and other seemingly little things that you have to deal with on a constant basis. You will always have to, but snow is one that can simply be eliminated. His response was almost immediate and unexpected, "You'd be a fool not to." I elaborated on my plans and told him that I would be making the adventure one of two ways; 1) with him 2) or by myself. The parental concern was evident on his face as he hesitantly agreed to the minimum 3 week excursion.

A few short weeks later, the '77 orange Matador was jammed to the roof with all of the worldly possessions I had collected throughout my lifetime. Also, along for the ride was my father's small suitcase. He was a simple, no frills kind of guy. There was no way to even see out the rear window, except for a mouse-hole sized tunnel through the back seat. This view ironically mirrored my newfound life philosophy of concentrating on where I was going, while occasionally looking over life lessons of the past, if only to avoid history repeating itself. I was looking forward to the trip as an opportunity to get to know my father on a deeper level. Up till this point we had a typical father-son relationship, with him providing guidance and mentoring. I wanted to know who he was outside of his fatherly role and duties. With him in the passenger seat only inches away I felt that the nature of our relationship was about to change.

Our first scheduled stop was in Columbia, Missouri at Steve's house. He was my next door neighbor in the college dorm for two years at Edinboro University, and had recently been diagnosed with cancer. Back in school, Steve was the one who entertained the entire dorm with his 100-watt stereo, as I previously mentioned. He liked to play it loud, not thinking twice when the walls would begin to vibrate. On more than one occasion, things literally fell off the shelves. The stereo had an old fashion 33 rpm turntable that stacked albums, dropping them one record at a time. The only problem was that he only owned three albums for the first two semesters. Fleetwood Mac, Steve Miller and Pink Floyd. He would let all three drop (one at a time) and play them. And flip them over – again and again. By the end of the first semester his neighbors had started a collection with the goal of purchasing additional albums for him to play.

Steve met us at the door. It took significant effort not to let out an audible gasp as the damage done since his diagnosis by this insidious disease was painfully obvious. His body had become emaciated and ashen in color, and his skin hung from his body, almost looking detached from his blood, bones and organs. This interaction brought back memories of the damage cancer had done to my mother. But this was different in the fact that it was my first experience with the potential death, and certain decline, of a peer. Somebody my age, in otherwise optimal health, surely couldn't have been invaded and his body surrendered to cancer this quickly. He had somehow been transformed from a chiseled, classically handsome young man to a gaunt shell of his former self. I did my best to put on a happy face, to cheer him up, but couldn't hide my concern. He did his best to be a cordial host and lighten the mood as we shared tales of life, and goings on, since college. We tried to avoid the elephant in the room, but we could only do so for so long. He recounted the progression and obvious ravages that cancer had taken. We talked into the darkness and he struggled to stay engaged and alert. He eventually fell asleep midsentence. I tucked him in with a pillow and a blanket and headed to my bed with a heavy heart.

The next morning, we delayed our departure waiting for Steve to get up. We said what I hoped would not be our final, tearful goodbyes. Dad and I waved and smiled as we pulled out of the driveway and headed down the road, but in the back of my mind I couldn't help but think about whether this would be the last time we'd meet in this life.

Three months later I learned of Steve's passing.

As I reflect back, I'm now grateful for my final time with him, as heavy as it was in the moment.

As we continued motoring Southwest, all the way through to Arizona. I turned to my co-pilot and mused, "Dad, as long as we are in the neighborhood, do you want to go see the Grand Canyon?". His response was something I truly did not expect. "Oh, that's just a big hole in the ground". It took a little convincing, but he eventually agreed, although reluctantly. It was a classic example of the overly practical lens that he looked at life through.

We arrived at the Grand Canyon at the crack of dawn, to a magnificent view, as the sun slowly rose above the canyon walls. Pulling into a parking spot on the north side of the canyon, I requested that my father go ahead and check out the wheelchair access and the quality of the view. While I remained behind, in the car waiting on my dad's canvassing efforts, I decided to enhance the experience by imbibing on some cannabis that I had stashed away.

We walked down the sidewalk toward the newly built observation deck. The trees separating the sidewalk from the edge of this enormous and remarkable wonder of nature eventually gave way to a surreal photo opportunity, with the canyon in the background. Since selfies were not to be invented for 30 years, I asked my dad to remain stationary while I went down the sidewalk to get just a little bit better location in front of the focus-pulling backdrop. Reaching the ideal spot, I popped the front end of my chair and positioned the footrest of my chair on top of a rock along the side of the path, for stability. After the obligatory serious pictures, along with some goofy snapshots, I casually backed off the rock. Before I knew it my rear wheel had slipped off the side of the path and I was rolling in slow motion toward the edge of the canyon.

The chair flipped, and as I lay on the ground noticing the edge of the canyon a mere few feet away, it became apparent how close I was to disaster. Almost as fast, I heard my father's footsteps as he ran toward me. Something I hadn't seen in 20 years. With the assistance of a couple tourists from Japan we quickly righted the ship, with the worry still deeply etched across my father's face. The rest of the day looking at the Canyon was relatively uneventful. We realized after that incident just how right and wrong my dad was about the Grand Canyon. It was just a hole in the ground, but even mere holes in the ground can cause grand disasters.

The next stop on the tour was another hole in the ground, as my father affectionately titled the wonders, called the Carlsbad caverns. He put up a mild resistance to visiting at first, but realized the effort was futile. As we slowly descended into the cavern, I noticed a divergence in the path ahead, with a sign pointing left that clearly read: "wheelchairs not advised beyond this point". Wanting to get the full exploring and spelunking experience for my money and knowing that my father would insist on the safer of the two passages, I quickly pointed to an interesting rock formation on the right and subtly steered my chair to the left. There is no mystery to my sense of adventure, even and especially after my accident. My adrenaline surged as the reason for the sign quickly became apparent. The path quickly became steeper and we rapidly descended further and further into the moist, dark cavern. The trip down was relatively quick and easy, but the return not so much.

The rock pathway was moist with dew as we both pushed with maximum effort, and the assistance of a couple of passersby. Thank goodness for kind, helpful strangers. The elements were stacking up and working against us. I glanced over my shoulder at the very reddened face of my father and realized the potential danger. If my father was to slip, trip or stroke out I would become folklore of the cavern.

You would think I'd have learned a lesson from the Grand Canyon incident. We both breathed a sigh of relief upon reaching the entrance. My father held back his anger as I confessed to my plan. That was the end of our sketchy adventures on that trip. It was the least I could do for my dad who had reluctantly agreed to this voyage in the first place; I wasn't helping to convince him that he had made the right choice.

The next stop was a little known town, Las Vegas, Nevada…

My father's first thought as we drove down the strip in Vegas: "I wonder what the electric bill must be for all the lights". On the other hand, I just sat back and enjoyed the show. Up until this point we had managed to stay in separate rooms, because along the way there were many nights when my father's snoring woke me up even from the room across the hall. But the sticker shock on the room prices in Las Vegas created an obligatory roommate situation for us over the next three days. The solution proved effective at exposing the generational divide.

On the first day, we headed out together and prioritized playing blackjack and slots, followed by dinner. He headed back to the room for the night shortly after that dinner wrapped up. The novelty and excitement of my first time in Vegas kept my adrenaline running. There was no stopping me, I was willing to try anything and everything the city had to offer. So I rode that adrenaline rush all the way to the slot machines and blackjack tables. Before I knew it, I was passing my father at the room in the early morning. If I had to guess it was sometime around 6 A.M., judging by the sun beginning it's climb into the sky. We shared a brief, rushed breakfast, and he headed out for the day as I headed to bed. I imagine he was creating his own adventure; a tamer version of what I was getting into. This behavioral pattern continued predictably over the next few days. As he would return to the room in the early evening, I was headed out for the night. We'd share our breakfast and I would punch in for the late, or early, shift, depending on how you orient your days, not to be seen again until first light.

After three days, we both agreed that we had made sufficient donations, both monetary and otherwise, to Sin City.

We left Vegas on a Friday, after I made one last trip down to the casino in a last ditch effort to recoup some of my losses. As I worked my way through the $20, I couldn't help but look forward, thinking about the day to come and what lie ahead for us. I was down to the last pull of that lever. Suddenly I was snapped back into the present, by fluorescent flashing lights and obnoxious ringing bells right in front of me. I had just spun three diamonds. What are the odds? Just like that, the extended pit stop in "Viva Las Vegas" was paid for. Not a bad return for one measly quarter.

By the time we got it all together and cashed out, we were Leaving town around 1 P.M. on a Friday, with a planned 4 hour stretch of open road ahead of us. We had no idea of what to expect, but after my lucky pull I was feeling pretty optimistic. By the end of the day we would be in the City of Angels, the farthest west either of us had ever been. An adventure to be sure.

As we turned off the I-10 and onto the 5, toward L.A., our initial West Coast culture shock was in full swing, due to the sheer chaotic energy of rush hour traffic. Up to this point, our experience with traffic jams had been 10 cars backed up at a light in Erie. And now we were looking at six lanes of freeway traffic pointing north and south, a total of a dozen lanes, with nobody moving so much as an eyebrow. It was 5 o'clock on a Friday afternoon. We weren't sure why they called it rush-hour traffic. Traffic had a mind of its own, and could sense when you were in a rush. You would get nowhere really fast.

After an eternity, we made it to Pasadena. Arrangements had been made to stay in the guest house on the property where Buck and his wife currently rented a house. Our accommodations in reality ended up being a small motorhome parked on the lot. And truth be told, that motorhome had seen better days, to put it mildly; it was overgrown with vegetation, among other things. As my father opened up the door to my new "home", we both jumped back as a big fat rat scurried across the floor. Or a small possum. Either way I wasn't ready for a pet, or a roommate. Again, I could see that all too frequent look of concern etched deeply on my father's face. I was beginning to think that was his default at this point. He was more than happy to get a room at a local hotel and reconvene the next morning.

In typical macho fashion, that next morning, we both tried to hold back the tears as I dropped my father at LAX early on a Sunday morning. Reality smacked me upside the back of the head as I got back to my new home. The farthest I had lived away from home was in college. And that was about 20 miles, if there was a construction detour. Now I was going to be 3000 miles away, as the crow flew, and unable to just stop by for a visit on any old weekend. Intensifying my anxiety, there was definite concern about leaving my father home alone without a support system or letting that fall on my brother, as he was the only one still living in the vicinity. Dad had recently lost his wife of 35 years. Retired from his job of almost 50 years. And most of his friends had basically drifted away, since they were couple, or mutual friends with my mother. Us kids think it was likely too painful of a reminder to be around people who were friends with her. These days you don't find commitment like that. It isn't "trendy". But it was my dad.

I had been caught completely by surprise when, in a recent conversation with him, he stated rather bluntly that he really didn't have anything for which to live anymore. "Dad, having just retired you now have all the time to do whatever you want. You can travel". To which he replied simply, "I had the opportunity to travel when I was in the Navy." That was that.

It was apparent that the Pasadena accommodations would be very temporary. My initial experience with Los Angeles was… too hot, too crowded, too dirty. Very different from Erie, in almost every way that could be measured. It was just too much for this small town boy. The following day I was off again on a three month journey up and down the California coast to look for a place to set up a more permanent shop. After what seemed like a fruitless, never ending search, I found myself finally landing in the orchard-laden town of San Jose. The valley full of fruit trees had long since been replaced by startups in a place now known as Silicon Valley, to everyone who does not live there, the tech capital of the world.

After my initial hesitancy to get back into any body of water, I decided to give it a go; I needed a sport, I had been an athlete my entire life. There were several other adaptive swimmers living in the area, and we formed the Waterwheels Swim Club. The team fit in with my newfound devotion to swimming, providing the opportunity for regular training along with stroke analysis and development. In order to further expand the sport of adaptive swimming, we developed Sink or Swim - the first ever international adaptive swim clinic and meet, with adaptive swimmers from around the world. All the swimmers met in Santa Clara, California. The event provided videotape stroke analysis by professional coaches, as well as race technique. The clinic also looked at the newly developing area of sports psychology and was able to procure a leading authority on the subject.

By this point, swim training was happening twice a day, in the early morning and evening. A good morning session began at 6 A.M. and continued until 9 A.M. Then the drill was to quickly and efficiently get out of the pool and head off to work. Three full, productive hours of training before work felt good. After a full day's work, it was customary to grab a quick dinner and head to evening practice. The time between practices was filled with a full-time job, working for an adaptive van conversion company, and in beginning development stages of a new van rental business.

Swim. Work. Eat. Swim. Sleep. Repeat. That was life, and it was shaping up nicely.

CHAPTER 4

GOT TO HAVE SEOUL: A WALK ON THE WALLED SIDE

The '88 Seoul Paralympics were fast approaching, and the training was reaching a crescendo. Race strategies were being finalized and competitors times from meets around the world were being collected and analyzed. Travel itineraries for the U.S. team were being coordinated. I had made the final cut to represent the United States.

The official U.S. team travel policy was for everybody to meet in New York City and fly together to and from the international competitions. The kicker was that everyone was required to dress in what was called Class A travel uniform, which consisted of dress slacks, and a blue blazer. There is a definite swell of pride when you don the red, white and blue, traveling as an official member of a large team, for the 1st time. Having traveled previously with various teams to countless meets, these uniform and travel policies had become cumbersome. The novelty had long since worn off. Traveling in a blazer with buttons getting caught in the wheels is irritating, to say the least. However, I had learned a few tricks over the years. It was an amazing coincidence just how many veteran team members had doctor's appointments that could only be scheduled for the day the team was slated to travel. Schedule conflicts like this could only be remedied by rebooking on a later flight. This hack helped to avoid having to travel with a cluster of 100 or more physically challenged athletes. Another upside - it was much easier to convince the flight crew to upgrade one individual to a first class seat, easing the boarding process for all parties.

I decided to also make arrangements for additional post competition travel. Personal travel. Sightseeing and exploration. Cultural immersion. I made it a goal to attempt to schedule side excursions to various locales in the neighborhood of the competition, whenever I traveled somewhere new for swimming.

The good thing about being a swimmer was that the equipment and uniform took up minimal packing space. The only required items were a Speedo, goggles and a towel. In a lesson learned from previous years of travel, space considerations needed to be made for team uniforms and swag acquired at the Games. Shuttling around too much stuff proved to be overwhelming, and extremely inconvenient. The ideal solution was to package it in a box after the competition and ship it home, or convince a team member to take it with them on their return trip, so I didn't need to lug everything around. The real challenge was converting the other luggage, including a sleeping bag, into a manageable form. Only after several attempts at test packing and repacking, trying to figure out how it was all going to fit in bags and on my chair, did the final configuration get set. The intent when traveling was to be self-contained, carrying only that which could be personally managed, so as not to have to rely on assistance from others. On a previous travel experience, assistance from a Good Samaritan turned into disaster when key pieces, including medication and my passport, got lost in the shuffle. The result was spending an entire day replacing the vital documents and medication; time which could have been spent sightseeing, or other touristy indulgences.

The final packing configuration included a sleeping bag, which was bungee corded to the underside of the chair seat, and suspended over a net catchall, which stretched from front to back. Hanging from the back of the chair, inches off the ground, and in between the wheels, was a square bag. Additionally, there was a jampacked backpack, hanging from the backrest. To round out the luggage, there was a 2-foot duffel bag, which sat on my lap, and a fanny pack which contained all important documents, strapped around my legs at the knees. Care had to be taken not to lean too far back when loaded up, to avoid falling backwards. If you can, picture a turtle belly up on its shell. Before my accident, I would never have predicted I would spend more than 15 minutes packing, or more than ½ of a run through to make sure all was in order.

The after competition travel itinerary intention was to make my way from Seoul, first to Hong Kong, followed by Beijing, Bangkok, Singapore and then to wrap it up, make my way for a bit of R&R, in Bali, Indonesia. The trip was scheduled to take four weeks after the conclusion of the competition, with a loose knit itinerary, intentionally.

The lack of detail provided the preferred flexibility to optimize unforeseen experiences wherever they appeared, and to decrease anxiety of trying to follow too exacting a schedule. There's a definite time and place for a plan, and post grueling international competition isn't one of them.

The competition at the '88 Seoul Paralympic Games was amazing, with the people of Seoul proving to be most gracious hosts. They were able to seamlessly transition between the Olympic Games and re-organize the competition and ceremonies sites, in only two short weeks following the Olympic Games. What hustle and bustle it must have been, but they remained composed and made it look effortless. All of the various venues were filled to capacity for the duration of the Paralympic games. All of the events were extremely well-attended with spectators and onlookers. Entering the Olympic Stadium for the opening ceremonies, with 108,000 people cheering wildly, was indescribable. The competition was top-notch, numerous Paralympic and International records were broken during the events. Unfortunately, none of those records belonged to me. My personal best finish throughout competition was fourth place in individual freestyle and fifth place in 25-meter butterfly and 100-meter freestyle respectively. I missed that podium by a few milliseconds, by what might as well have been a month.

But, just as life had been up to that point, not all of the experience was fun and games. The swimming portion of the Games was well under way, and we were approaching the butterfly segment of the competition. My best stroke.

Prior to the event I was approached by one of my teammates, Scott, who had a worried look on his face. He confessed that he had significant concerns over the upcoming 25-meter butterfly and his lack of experience swimming it on the international level. His specific concern was the difference in distance between the familiar domestic distance of 25 yards and the international standard of 25 meters. His only butterfly experience was swimming 25 yards in the U.S. The way the quadriplegic class of swimmers approached the 25 meter distance was to take one deep breath at the start and then bury your head, covering the entire distance of that race in one breath. It was the most efficient, and fastest, way to swim the distance because to rise up for a breath without a leg kick significantly affected forward momentum, especially for a quad. However, by the end of the race, oxygen in a racer's lungs was always completely depleted.

I reassured Scott that I had personally done the meter distance numerous times successfully and concluded with the phrase "I guarantee that you **will** be able to make the distance. Besides, what's the worst that can happen? Even if you run out of breath you can always come up for air. But simply put, if you come up for a breath, you lose."

Scott was scheduled to swim in the heat prior to mine, so I was on the starting end of the pool watching with his mom. *BANG!* The starter's pistol for the race went off. Scott started strong and was battling back and forth with the leaders. We were at the starting end of the pool cheering wildly. The good news was that he was able to make the distance with only one breath and managed to finish in 2nd place. As I watched him reach for the side of the pool to lift up for that all-important first breath his hand slipped and just as he started the big inhale, his face slipped back underneath the water. He was gassed from the intensity of the race, and couldn't get himself up to break the waterline again.

In all the confusion of the race finish, with timers, officials and lifters all over at that end of the deck, buzzing and hurrying, he went momentarily unnoticed except by his mother and I. We were frantically trying to get someone at the other end of the pool to notice his situation and get his face above water. As they came to lift him out of the pool, they realized what had happened and he was immediately pulled onto the deck with his legs bent at the knees, hanging over the side. They began CPR by alternating chest compressions with breaths. After what seemed like an eternity, we noticed his legs began to shake, which was a good sign indicating that he had literally come back to life. We saw each other several times over the ensuing years and our conversation always greeted each other with that ominous phrase, "What's the worst thing that can happen?". He recovered over the next three days in Seoul General Hospital, and his Paralympic Games in Seoul were finished. It was déjà vu for me, but on the other side of the story. That didn't make it any less terrifying in the moment.

After the closing ceremonies for the games, the athlete village cleared out quickly, with everybody returning to their respective countries and various, busy lives. I traveled with the rest of the US team via bus to the airport in Seoul. As we arrived at the airport, I could feel my anxiety level rising pretty rapidly. This was the point where I was scheduled to split from the rest of the team and start my most extensive after competition travel to date. Solo to boot. As the rest of the team prepared to board a flight for New York city, I was off to find Singapore Airlines for a flight to Hong Kong. As much as I tried to imagine traveling in a foreign country where English is uncommon and spoken primarily by businesspeople, it quickly became apparent that there were going to be some awkward communication issues. But, luckily for the duration of my time, there was usually somebody available to interpret.

The first stop on my Asian adventure was Hong Kong. I had read about the city and its hustling and bustling nature, but was not prepared for the reality. As the flight approached the runway tarmac in Hong Kong, the view of the city reminded me of the pop-up pages in a children's book. Or maybe a 3-D greeting card perhaps. Over the next few days, I made several trips into the city and was amazed at the numbers of skyscrapers crammed within such close proximity, and the sheer amounts of people everywhere, no matter what time of day it was. There was no space, for anything. Every one of them in a hurry, and with me in tourist mode, it almost felt like I was being overrun. I'm not sure whether it's their hustling lifestyle, my relatively slow pace or low line of vision, but I met numerous "people" up close and personal as they ran me over. I even had one end up directly in my lap. While in the city, I sampled several unique culinary experiences, wanting to expose my Western pallet to the local fare. The biggest concern being that I hoped the delicacies, some of which I still have not identified a full three decades later, would agree with my unsophisticated gastrointestinal requirements. This created a quadriplegic traveler's potentially worst nightmare – toileting needs are often more immediate and sensitive in nature for us.

Next up: Beijing. The flight departing from Hong Kong was on China Airlines. This was back in the days where it was legal to smoke on an airplane, in a hospital, or wherever the addiction reared it's head. During this flight the majority of passengers were smokers, with the smoke so thick that it was difficult to see across the aisle. A complementary in-flight, foul-smelling, dense fog. Another peculiarity observed in flying through that hemisphere was that passengers take all kinds of unique carry-on items, as evidenced by child's bikes and trikes, a lamp and a chicken in a cage, to name just a few. Here, you are nickel and dimed for carry-ons. Judging by their items, it was a free-for-all, although I'm not sure how that has changed in more recent years. There were several instances where limited overhead bin space turned into a heated confrontation, and in one instance hand-to-hand combat. Eventually, everything settled down and we were able to take off.

Everyone that has ever flown has heard, and promptly ignored, the safety precaution message at the beginning of the flight: "be careful in opening overhead bin, as the contents may have shifted in flight". This flight was a poster example of why that particular warning exists. As I sat daydreaming and observing all the activity, looking through the haze across the aisle, I happened to notice a man stand and begin to unlatch the overhead bin. The door forcefully sprung open, due to that content shifting that they warned you about, and out tumbled a 2' x 3' framed picture, which proceeded to fall corner first square on the head of the unsuspecting woman sitting underneath it. She was immediately knocked unconscious. Needless to say, the scene was somewhat chaotic. When we arrived in Beijing the flight was met by a team of paramedics, and the woman was carried away immediately on a gurney.

After departing the plane, I caught the shuttle to the Americana Hotel, which I don't believe still exists in modern day Beijing. It was located in the outskirts of downtown Beijing. This lodging accommodation had the reputation of having a westernized environment. As we travelled down the road, I noticed that the vast majority of the afternoon rush hour traffic jam consisted of bicycles, with the occupants dressed in regional clothing, which is a bit more ornate and complex than traditional western garments. It caused a flash back, affectionately and a tad ironically, to the portion of the cross country trip from Las Vegas to Pasadena at 5 o'clock on a Friday afternoon. Only this rush hour consisted of bicycles instead of cars, and a more uniform dress code. I was clearly tired, and long overdue for rest to refresh the mind. The extended, arduous days' worth of travel made sleep easy to come by that night.

Upon waking up on my first full day in Beijing, the plan was to head to the infamous Tiananmen Square. Travel through downtown Beijing in a wheelchair was difficult and more than a bit bumpy due to the cobbled brick sidewalk and street. Additionally, the sheer numbers of bicycles and people going every which way made for an even more challenging sightseeing experience. While pushing down the road that ran past the Great Hall, it helped me to reminisce on the familiar façade portrayed in government controlled newsfeeds during the heinous Tiananmen massacre. This was only a few months prior to the People's revolt in Tiananmen Square, in which hundreds of people were killed by the military, who were simply sent in for crowd control. During the ensuing years, on several occasions, I have thought back to passing by the People's Hall, and mentally superimposing the now famous picture of the lone individual in the road staring down and stopping a tank that was just feet away, into that scene as I saw it in peacetime.

During the time I spent traveling about Beijing, I couldn't help but notice that I was getting more than your average number of strange and inquisitive looks. In talking to the locals, their suggested reasoning for all the looks I received was the way that Chinese people viewed and handled spinal cord injury, and disabilities in general. The medical community would stabilize the individual and give them back to their family, who were told to take them home and make them comfortable for whatever their remaining stay on earth may be. Without the benefit of today's modern medicine and rehabilitation techniques, there was very little the families could do. So, as a result, the Chinese people rarely experienced someone in a wheelchair in public, experiencing their culture and doing things independently, much less some random goofy-looking white dude.

Another day's adventure took me to the Forbidden City, and I quickly realized the loaded meaning behind the word forbidden - at least from a wheelchair traveler's point of view. The Chinese people believe very seriously in spirits. These spirits are said to travel around the city, existing among the living, going wherever they want. However, according to several different sources, are unable to lift their feet and thus have no choice but to shuffle as they walk. One way to limit spirit travel into the Forbidden City, was to put down a 8" x 8" beam across the doorway, and the main entrance to the city, thus keeping the shuffling spirits out. Those of us travelling in wheelchairs, or using alternative methods, were collateral sacrifices. It eventually required a four person team to lift me over the beam, in order to get inside. The "team" that assisted me so that I could experience the Forbidden City had become a metaphor akin to "taking a village" – although I was just starting to realize, and appreciate, how true it really was. It may be hard to believe, but this was going to prove to not be the biggest obstacle in the Forbidden City for me.

After spending the day checking out the various buildings in the area, an impending intestinal urge had taken over top priority, and was at the forefront of the 'to-do immediately' list. The need to find a bathroom, and fast, was increasing exponentially. With each passing moment, I inched closer to critical mass. Locating the necessary facilities was slowed down by the language barrier and lack of ability to interpret signage, as it was mostly Chinese characters, with no alternative translations. So, in my best broken sign language, more affectionately known as hand signals, I asked locals where to go, literally. Upon entering the restroom, I looked around and noticed a critical component was missing from the scene. It quickly became apparent that there were no traditional western commode-style porcelain toilets upon which to sit. The only option available were areas with the outlines of 2 feet and between them an 8-ish inch round hole in which to make a deposit. This was a major detail that had been missed in the extensive trip preparations. Unfortunately, no one had informed me that the custom in relieving oneself here was to put your feet within the designated outlines on the floor, drop your drawers, squat, and relieve.

Needless to say, this was going to be difficult, or next to impossible for me to execute. Everything was compounded by the urgent nature of this side trip. This may have been where they got the phrase, "necessity is the mother of invention". This was the day that I developed what would prove to be an invaluable technique. One that I was able to fall back on in future situations to relieve myself, while in a wheelchair and seemingly without proper accommodations. This happens more often than you would think. When in a bind, I wouldn't need to stress anymore. This technique involved placing the chair over the hole and using the chair's calf strap as a sling under my thighs, on which to sit. This newly developed skill served me well on several camping trips over the ensuing years. To save the faint of heart, I won't go into detail but if we ever get a chance to talk in person, I would be willing to fill in the blanks. I got several perplexed looks from passersby, as you can imagine, and probably would have done yourself if you happened upon the scene. The other minor detail I forgot to mention was that there were no stalls or dividers, and people were surely not shy about looking as they strolled on by.

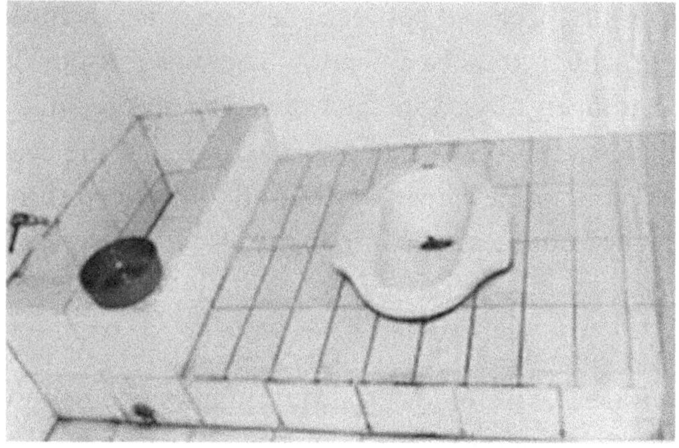

The last day in Beijing included a much-anticipated trip to the Great Wall. So let's briefly rewind. Prior to leaving the United States, I had exclaimed to my friend that while in China, I was going to ride a wheelie on the Great Wall. As anticipated, he looked at me right then with an all too familiar, sarcastic, and skeptical look and exclaimed, "Yeah, right!" As we arrived at the Great Wall, the theme of inaccessibility once again took center stage. Sitting at the base, I dejectedly stared at the first of the 42 steps that stood between me and the top of the wall. Those steps might as well have been the distance from Earth to Jupiter. I sighed and said, "oh darn", or maybe a somewhat less PG version of that phrase out of sheer frustration. Just then, I heard a voice to my left, asking "what's wrong?". After explaining my desire to get up on the Great Wall, we parted ways and I continued my tour of the structure, reading plaques and taking in the immenseness that was the Wall, at its base. Even that limited view was largely enamoring.

All of a sudden, I noticed that I was being surrounded by five individuals. Unsure what was happening, they began to grab and lift my chair in unison and suddenly I understood. The next thing I knew, I was being carried up the stairs, all the way to the top. I was amazed that one individual took it upon himself to organize others to help make a stranger's wish come true. Collectivist cultural values showed their true colors.

Once on top of the wall, I found the surface is amazingly flat, enabling me to easily push, almost gliding, for miles to take in the enormity of the structure. The wall literally went on for hundreds of miles and faded into the countryside, with breathtaking vistas. Explaining it is not even close to the same as experiencing it. I finished the day on a high from all the beauty and sheer enormity, and as I rolled back to the entry point, a voice inside my head said, "this is the place". Just ahead lay a gentle downslope about 30 yards long. I recruited a nearby man, as I approached, and with the assistance of several unofficial interpreters got my point across to him. His task was to go to the end of the gentle downslope with my camera and, when I nodded my head, snap a picture. With a puzzled look on his face, understandably so, he took his position with a bit of reluctance. I leaned back and began to ride a wheelie down the slope, nodded my head and he captured the moment with my camera. This was back in the days where a roll of film that had been used needed to be taken to the drug store, developed, and then hope the pictures turned out. Unlike today where you get instantaneous digital results. So, it would be one month before I knew the results and if our efforts were fruitful.

Upon returning home, the film was taken out for development, as it had become a top priority for me. Retrieving the photos from the drug store, the first order of business was to locate all the Beijing pictures. Of course, they were in the last envelope in which we looked. The resulting picture from the top of the wall turned out even better than expected and gave me the idea of turning the picture into a Christmas postcard with the phrase "Greetings from the Great Wall of China". Included in this newly established seasonal mailing list was my friend Mike, who if you remember had his doubts. The cards were mailed out, and a week later, I received a phone call, before caller ID. The voice on the other end of the now-obsolete receiver barked, "you son of a bitch, I can't believe you did it!"

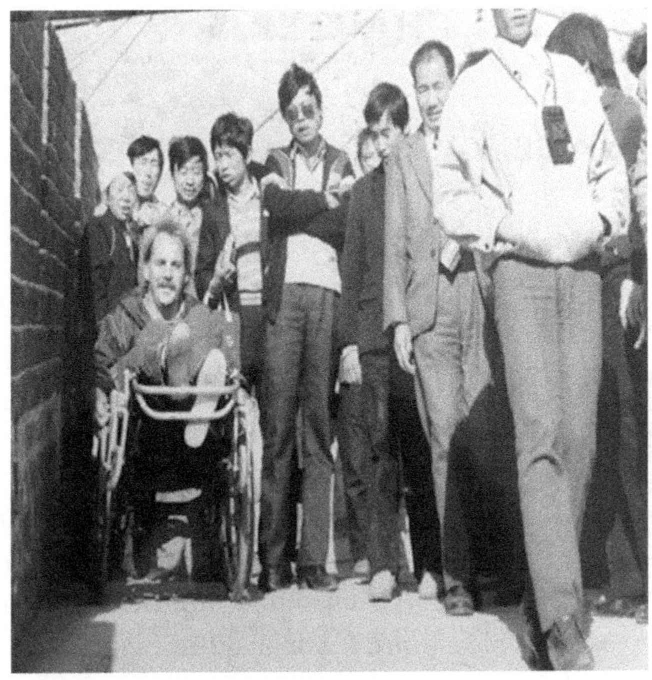

(Greetings from the Great Wall of China, Dec '88)

CHAPTER 5

BASEBALL TOUR DE JOUR

Flashback to the early '60s:

As the oversize green metal doors that lead to the field opened, I was overwhelmed at the site before me. There, before my tiny body and oversized eyes, lay a huge vibrant green field of grass, perfectly manicured, surrounding a deep brown infield, dotted by four bright white bases. Thousands of orange seats surrounded the field. We were a group of 7 year olds from a regional Little League attending our first major league baseball game at the cavernous Cleveland Municipal Stadium. All we could think to say was, "WOW". Immediately followed by a cartoonish series of jaws hitting the floor. The parents who were chaperoning the group tried to act like they were unimpressed, but you could see the twinkle in their eyes as they flashed back to their childhood. It was an awe-inspiring scene.

We were some of the first people there joining the field crew and players warming up with a casual game of toss, and batting practice. I immediately ran down the stairs with the sound of my dad yelling after me to be careful, and don't get out of sight, or something like that. That wasn't where my focus was at the moment. Straight down to the railing we scurried, to stand in amazement as our heroes Jim Perry, Early Wynn, and Mudcat Grant stood a mere few feet away. There stood the real life embodiment of the players whose faces decorated the front side of the baseball cards that sat neatly tucked away in a mounting shoebox collection under my bed. Some of my most prized possessions to date. My weekly allowance investment that came packaged with a flat, dried out piece of bubblegum that immediately shattered into shards upon impact with teeth. The real investment was never the gum, but the accompanying card.

From that first game, I had thought about how this same game was being played 162 times a year by 18 other teams (now, a total of 30 teams). I wondered if the other teams and stadiums were as wonderful. Perhaps one day in the future I'll be able to travel to another park. Or maybe two.

Fast forward 42 years, and that childhood dream was now becoming reality. The van was in drive and so was my anticipation of the upcoming cross country tour to visit all of the major league baseball parks in the same season. This was going to be the fulfillment of a childhood dream since the age of 7.

While preparing for the journey there were several offers with people wanting to join in the excursion. Some out of safety concerns and others because of the cool nature of the adventure. But the decision was made to go it solo, and push the limits of a quad travelling alone. I like to think I had long since perfected the art of travelling, for various purposes, to different destinations. I had long held the belief that traveling solo had its benefits. The theory being that if you're traveling alone and want to talk to someone, you're forced to reach out and make contact with someone brand new, the potential for infinite new friends and varied connections. Otherwise, if you're travelling with someone you know the tendency is to converse with the familiar partner. The plans did include passengers, like my wife, daughter and big brother to name a few, for various, brief segments of the trip. The decision was made to go it solo on this trip with dad as my now spiritual co-pilot; the person who had lit this baseball tour fire many years ago.

I had to make the following planning considerations:

- Time frame
  - How much time did I have to dedicate to this trip?
  - How many parks did I want to visit? All of them? A certain number?
  - What pace did I want to travel? For speed or leisure, or a mix?
  - Did I have any other objectives on this trip? Sites, and sights, aside from parks that I wanted to take in? Any people that I wanted to rendezvous with?
- Geography
  - What area did I want to visit? Any areas I wanted to avoid, or would need to consider alternative travel methods?
- Each team's schedule
  - Visit each team's website
- Putting the pieces of the scheduling puzzle together
  - Again, square pegs + round holes

Other considerations

- Finding tickets
  - When to purchase these tickets?
  - From who?
  - First option: call parks ticket office directly
    - This provides most direct, best, cheapest and most accessible seat options.
  - Second option: Online ticket sales
    - Stubhub for re-sale
  - Third option: Day of game sales
    - Scalpers
    - Box office, in person for standby
- Accessibility
  - Older parks have ambience and rich baseball history
  - Accessibility definitely an afterthought
  - Accommodations are usually possible, as long as you give as much advanced notice as possible
  - Occasionally accessible seating is not available to the general public
    - A small perk
  - The newer the facility the better
    - Specifically parks built since 1992
  - In between
    - Usually they have incorporated the ADA regulation of providing a minimum number of accessible seats at each price level
    - The longer you wait, the more likely the tickets you get are at the back of the section

- ○ Older stadiums
  - ▪ Parks built earlier on, and not since modified almost always only offer accessible seats at the back of each section
- Housing
  - ○ Tentative and tight schedule
  - ○ Didn't want to reserve hotel rooms
  - ○ Potential for car-camping
  - ○ Made accommodations through: the internet, info/chain numbers, friends, family and kind strangers (word of mouth)
- Timing
  - ○ Coordination between logical geographical progression and team schedules
  - ○ Too tight of a schedule would ensure an unforeseen kink
  - ○ Still needed a general plan of action

Months had been spent working out the details of this summer-long excursion. The complexity of the route and seemingly natural sequence of stadiums to be visited was magnified due to the variety of the team's home schedules. They weren't working on my schedule, that's for sure. The logical geographic sequence of stops was often interrupted because a particular team was on the road during the given time that I was due to be in that region. Also, there was a requisite need for flexibility on a trip of this nature, and that required the creative combination of a variety of transportation modes being employed. Planes, trains, automobiles, and a couple buses were used at different points throughout the trip.

The 2001 Honda Odyssey, that had faithfully taken me where I needed to go for years, was consciously organized with all the equipment necessary to support this month long portion of the journey. The most critical items were placed within arm's reach, in order to avoid needless delays where I need to stop and climb into the back, dismantling all that had been carefully packed. There was just enough room left behind the drivers' seat to squeeze my chair in after transferring to the cockpit seat. The plan was to only stop for refueling and brief, necessary stops.

Ever since attending my first major league game at the now defunct Cleveland Municipal Stadium, that had been demolished in early '97, I sat wondering if all the parks in the majors were as majestic as the lush vibrant green field, with crisp uniforms on larger than life players.

An hour later the van was set to cruise control and easily winding though the Sierra Nevada mountains with whisps of clouds clinging to the tops of the trees like cotton balls suspended in the sky. Donner Lake sat quietly in the valley below. Surrounded by a lush green carpet of treetops, taking in this sight caused my spirits to soar. A gentle breeze floated above the rippled water that was sparkling pristinely in the sunshine. Somehow, they felt interconnected, yet completely independent, simultaneously. The euphoric feeling that had taken up residence in me, and the anticipation of summer-long adventures to come as I wove through the majestic mountain scenery, soon gave way to long desolate patches of seemingly endless desert. I had known that the first day would hold the biggest surge of energy. Based on that, I decided to extend the driving distance and see how far I could make it before that initial burst faded. After a brief 17-hour cruise, I reached my first nights' stay, just outside of Denver. The mile-high city. This was the only hotel room reserved in advance on the trip. The uncertainty of what each day would bring and needing flexibility to modify driving distance helped me be at ease with that decision. On any given day flexibility was essential.

I had known lodging would be a concern for me, since I was unfamiliar with more than a handful of the cities I was to be visiting. I was no stranger to traveling, but many of these specific regions were brand new. Unsure of what to expect, or whether there would be availability, made it bit of a riskier adventure. Each day was thrilling, nonetheless.

The first park on the journey was Coors Field, which sits nestled in downtown Denver. Not coincidentally the opponent in the first game on the trip happened to be the San Francisco Giants; my home team. I was excited to get to watch them play in a new environment. With game time still 5 hours away, there was plenty of time to connect with an old friend of mine who lived locally. From there we could circumnavigate the neighborhood surrounding the park, and then enjoy a crisp evening at the ballpark together.

Part of the plan on the tour was to incorporate regular exercise. The idea was to push the neighborhoods around each park, getting a feel for each city. I wanted to truly experience the unique traditions of the local fans and sample the local cuisine, like the infamous brats in Milwaukee. At every park, I hoped to cruise the exterior of each park to see how each city partook in tailgating; one of my favorite activities that customarily accompanied America's pastime. Once inside, we took time to check out the nooks and crannies of the park's interior, meeting and interacting with local fans. Each group seemed to have their own unique brand of fanaticism.

Also, I had made sure to stow away a hand cycle in the van, not wanting to interrupt my training schedule and to utilize when necessary to get around, intending to experience each location to the fullest during the tour. I knew it would be a whirlwind. When planning, I hesitated when deciding whether to include the cumbersome bike, as it took up more than its fair share of space in the back. And I wasn't sure when, or if, I would need double up and use the van as a bedroom. It was ultimately decided that the money saved by staying in the Odyssey would not outweigh the benefit of getting a full night's rest in a hotel with a real bed, clean sheets and pillows.

The tour continued east toward the geographical heart of American baseball, in Kansas City and St. Louis. Upon leaving Kauffman stadium after the second game on my tour, the first scheduling challenge quickly presented itself unannounced. There had been unforeseen circumstances that lead to inevitable delays, causing my arrival in Kansas City to line up exactly with game time and first pitch. Since I was in such a hurry, I didn't get a chance to reserve a hotel room before the game started. I found myself in a bind at 10pm, with no place to sleep after the game ended, and bedtime speedily approaching for this middle-aged man. The thought of locating an accessible and acceptable room and climbing in and out of the van to check availability, after the day I already had, seemed like a daunting task. After dejectedly climbing back into the van after a third "no vacancy" in a row, I stared into the night and pondered the situation.

Then all of the sudden the answer appeared right before my very eyes. My weary eyes focused in on a billboard, with all of the surrounding vegetation magically falling away. *1 (800) 4CHOICE.* It was so obvious, why had I not thought of this? With one flip of my cell phone, a call was made, and I was able to be connected to a nationwide system of available hotel rooms. It quickly became a habit on the road to stop mid afternoon, estimate where the end location would be for the day, and reserve a hotel room by simply telling them where I was travelling and asking what was available in that area. Amazing how far technology had brought us.

Another of the planning challenges came to the fore front after pointing the van south toward the next park. Ideally, the next logical and convenient stop would have been in Texas for two games. It turned out that only one of the teams was in town, and it was not feasible to wait for the other to return. Texas would require a separate flight to the area later in the summer. So, instead it was a quick overnight in the French Quarter. Beignets and coffee at Café DuMonde, in the morning and on the way to a date at Tropicana Field in Tampa.

After a game at the Trop the next morning's agenda included house cleaning. The plan was to clean and organize the van. Only after the van was spotless, I would swing by the airport and pick up my wife and daughter so they could join me for the East Coast segment of the trip. For some mysterious reason, the girls did not share my desire to drive back and forth across the entire United States but wanted to share part of the trip. The part that got them a little bit of baseball, and a lot of reconnecting with family. Our family was, and still is, predominantly based on the East Coast, so it also provided the opportunity to visit my Mother-in-Law in Ocala. Since there were a couple days before the next scheduled game in Miami, the girls had requested a side trip to Key West. Although adding an additional 400 miles onto the trip wasn't part of the original plan, this segment was now a family vacation.

After a game in the muggy summer air of Miami, the next logistical complication in the tour arose. Although the teams in the northeast were more geographically proximal at this point, the question remained: would they have a home game schedule during a realistic time frame? Unfortunately, the Baltimore Orioles were set to start an extended road trip the following week. So, in order to fit the Orioles into the schedule it required me rising at the crack of dawn and driving to the airport for a day trip to Baltimore. A couple of phone calls to the transportation authority the previous day provided the accessible bus route that would drop me off at the front gates to the park. Although this was an inconvenient side trip, there was an upside. The Orioles were playing an inter-league game against my San Francisco Giants. What are the odds. And because the prior nights game had been rained out, they were playing a double header. Double bonus. Although quite weary by the time my head hit the pillow back in Florida, the day gave a glimpse into the modern day professional athletes hectic lifestyles. They somehow managed to do all this travel and still perform. All the while away from their families and loved ones. The girls had spent a casual day with Nana, or as my wife called her, Mom. Included on their itinerary: shopping, spa treatments with a side trip to Busch Gardens. The height of luxury.

Once reunited with the girls, we continued our trip up the East Coast, next to Atlanta, for a Braves game. Again, they were uninterested in watching the Braves, and instead chose to spend time shopping in the Underground.

Upon arrival in Pennsylvania, I was to exchange my current traveling partners. My wife and daughter ended their time on the road with me, stopping to spend time with my brother-in-law and his family. My wife and I were both raised in PA. Her brother had stayed in the area, outside of Philadelphia, to raise his kids. My brother came over from Erie to join me on my road travels. After a family outing, all of us going to see the Phils, my older sibling would be copiloting for the ballparks of the northeast. Together we would make it to seven parks in eight days. Included on the list were the two New York teams; a Friday night affair between the rival Mets and Yankees in the Bronx. Due to the anticipated popularity of this game it was one of the few advance purchase tickets. After fighting crosstown NYC traffic from Brooklyn to the Bronx, we made it to Yankee Stadium with plenty of time to spare till first pitch. This wasn't a feeling I was used to. We entered the park early to check out the history of the stadium, with a heavy mist hanging in the air. Shortly thereafter a light rain had begun and turned into a steady downpour. Then came the words we dreaded, "ladies and gentlemen, tonight's contest between the New York Mets and your New York Yankees has been postponed". Not only would we miss this unique opportunity to see these cross town rivals, but it would necessitate a separate return trip to the Big Apple at a later date. Unfortunately, the schedule dictated that the next day we were to be in Toronto for a game featuring the Blue Jays, so we promptly left Yankee Stadium and drove into the night.

Another difficult ticket to come by on the trip was to catch the Red Sox at Fenway. Since that portion of the trip was touch and go, the choice was made to purchase day of game seats at the park. These tickets are put up for sale two hours prior to the start time of the game, although if you wait until that point to line up for the tickets you are more than likely going to be out of luck. We lined up over three hours prior to game time and had been waiting for a little while when I was approached by park employees and directed to the ticket window that handles accessible seating. Although I was moments too late to score accessible seats on the Green Monster, we did manage to get tickets directly behind Pesky's Pole. They were close enough to read many of the signatures which had been added over the years. What a unique experience.

I considered the ease of scoring tickets to any venue as existing on a spectrum; most falling in the middle, but there was a range from very easy to next to impossible. On the other end of this spectrum was procuring tickets to a Montreal Expos game, now the Washington Nationals. With the Expo management having announced the sale and transplant of the team two years prior, only the most loyal of fans continued to show up. The guesstimated attendance was 1200 in the cavernous Olympic Stadium on the night we went. It was the quietest game I've ever attended. And that included my own little league games growing up in Erie. To prove the point, I sat along the 1st base line and my brother along 3rd base line, and we were able to carry on an only slightly elevated conversation. My brother and I parted ways after a game in Cleveland, watching the team that we spent our childhood rooting for.

The van was now pointed west and headed for home, having completed the major driving portion of the trip.

But, along the way there were the final four stops. The highlight of this portion was a Fourth of July contest between the Cubs and White Sox at Wrigley Field. The day included fireworks on the field with a bottom of the 9th winning run. What's more, this was followed by a citywide fireworks display, spanning the various boroughs as viewed from the upper level of this venerable park. I had pre-purchased two tickets for this game with the hopes of meeting a longtime friend of 30 years. I was disappointed when he cancelled morning of, due to a family emergency, but it opened up the possibility to scalp my ticket for an amount which covered the cost of both. I also understand family emergencies wait for no baseball excursion. A stop at Milwaukee between the games with the Cubs and White Sox yielded the best hot dog of the trip. Technically, yes, it was a sausage, but it was still by far and away the best.

Due to the limited time frame and more importance on seeing all the parks that summer, I did not do as much sightseeing as planned. I had set a time frame, but it was very much dictated by the schedule of the home games and the desire to avoid doubling back, like I did in flying to Baltimore. Generally, costs could be cut here and there by expanding the time frame and utilizing modern technology. The advice I would give is to be aware of potential snafus, such as rainouts, game scheduling conflicts, and other delays. Mitigate where you can but soak it all in otherwise. Don't sweat the small, inevitable changes of course. Over the span of this trip, I visited 30 parks in total, drove over 11,000 miles in a mere 6 weeks' time, and flew 15,000 miles – but I completed the journey, and enjoyed the entirety of it. Even the unforeseen speed bumps. I intentionally avoided too tight of a schedule, and still had to reschedule, but that's the beauty of baseball, the unpredictability.

If anyone is interested in my opinions on "bests" from different categories, food, experience, views, competition and otherwise: I would have to say the best "old school" ballpark was Fenway, for its originality, best "new school" park was Pac Bell (now Oracle) park for it's location right on the water (although I might be a tad biased there), the best accessibility was in Atlanta at the Braves stadium, and the best hot dog, which was actually a brat was found in Milwaukee.

The order that I took in each team and stadium went like this: Giants, Rockies, Royals, Cardinals, Devil Rays, Marlins, Orioles, Braves, Phillies, Yankees, Expos, Mets, Blue Jays, Indians, Pirates, Reds, Cubs, Brewers, Mariners, White Sox, Twins, Tigers, Rangers, Astros, A's, Diamondbacks, Dodgers, Angels, Padres.

The Angels game was bittersweet because it was the site of where the Giants had lost the World Series in 2002, and it was still too recent of a loss for this fan.

It was the trip of a lifetime for a baseball guy, and one that I highly recommend to celebrate and partake in America's pastime, and a sport that never goes out of style.

CHAPTER 6

FREE FALLING —
PART 1 — "BOING"

A group of us gathered at the great Shoreline Amphitheater, located in Mountain View, California. A reunion of friends, a large crane, and possibly, a severe lack of common sense; what could go wrong?

The intent was simply to let a stranger strap us in, let the bungee cords and gravity do their jobs, giving us the ultimate adrenaline rush. The bungee cords were calculated for each of our weights, and hopefully still elastic as ever. From there we were loaded in a basket and lifted to the top of the 200-foot crane and jump. Launch ourselves off the edge and towards the pavement, the thrill of a lifetime for most. It could be said that this was a typical day out, except that everyone in the group was a quadriplegic with varying degrees of paralysis from the chest down. All of us utilized a wheelchair for everyday mobility. Needless to say, we attracted some attention from the crowd that had gathered to observe at the base of the crane.

The ground crew consisted only of two people. One individual in charge of strapping people in, and the other to run the crane. A good friend of mine for many years,

Richard C. was the first victim, or participant, depending how you look at it. He was loaded in the basket and raised up to the top of the crane to the position predetermined for him. From the ground, we watched as he was assisting in slowly inching himself to the edge, to the final jumping position, his legs bent at the knees, hanging over the side. With the crowd starting the countdown backwards from ten, when it got to zero, he nodded his head and the next thing any of us realized, he was speeding towards the ground at an alarming speed. The bungee eventually tightened, and we breathed a collective sigh of relief, he paused momentarily mid-air, then he changed directions, being propelled away from Earth. This was equally as shocking to witness. The pattern repeated several times. He finally, yet too quickly came to a rest. His hair was shooting off in every direction imaginable, almost like he was a kid who had stuck a knife in a socket.

Next up? The other Richard. That would be me. I was given the choice of strapping my two lower limbs together for additional control and support during the bungee. However, I declined, thinking that they would go into immediate spasm, from the excitement, and remain stiff throughout the jump. This sounds simply inconvenient, but it's much more than that when you deal with spasms and other lower limb loss of control every single day. The harness had four straps, two on each leg, extending around the shoulders, all converging just above the waist, as the point of attachment for the bungee. Transferring over to the edge of the basket, the adrenaline started to course through me, while the final strap and other checks were performed. Still, I put on a brave face, that was fueled by equal parts testosterone and adrenaline. I was then kindly assisted in my transfer to the basket. The next, immediate instructions were to sit on the edge of the basket for the duration of the ride to the top of the monstrous crane; a direct correlation between my excitement, which eventually gave way to anxiety, and our distance from the ground. As the basket slowed to a stop, the once familiar faces on the ground became smaller and smaller, until they became indistinguishable. The venue had chosen to store a traffic sign nearby with an accessibility logo, ironically placed directly below the jumping area. It was either an ominous sign or warning, which one was yet to be determined. I heard the faint countdown from below, "three – two – one – JUMP!". Hesitating briefly, I then obliged the crowd down below, and scooted off the edge to meet my fate.

The free fall was tremendously exciting, with familiar faces coming in and out of focus. I could feel the bungees begin to tighten, halting my plummet, and beginning to send me in reverse, mere feet from the ground. The straps squeezed the legs that I had chosen not to secure, which then went in different directions much to my dismay. Paradoxically, I was able to control my upper body. I realized, in the rush to take my turn, I had forgotten to empty my bladder. As you could probably predict, this turned out to be problematic, the straps constricting in just the wrong spot. The pressure proved to be too much, and my overly full bladder let loose with each successive contraction of the cords. The people on the ground, going in and out of focus, began to point at the sudden appearance of a mysterious liquid in the sky on a sunny day. I could see several individuals pointing at the freefalling liquid with questions on their face as to its etiology. Suddenly two and two were put together, and I watched as the group scattered away from the landing site. The golden shower gently fell to earth. Before the ride came to its conclusion, I heard someone in the crowd call out my soon-to-be new nickname, "Hey, Rainman". Equal parts excitement and embarrassment simultaneously palpably coursed through my body.

FREE FALLING, PART TWO: "LOOPY"

Flashback to my 20's:

A warm breeze flowed through the slightly cracked window in my light orange AMC Matador. It was mid-morning on what was forecast to be a warm day in the valley, as I left the Los Angeles area, where I was currently residing, and wound through the surrounding mountains. I was on a mission to meet Peter, and go stunt-planing that afternoon. The word was that he was a former Bush pilot, flying missions in and out of Central America. He was said to be able to land a plane on a runway the size of a football field and, since moving back to the United States, had taken up the lucrative hobby of stunt-planing. Tricks to be included in the day's lesson: barrel rolls, loop-the-loop, fully-inverted, and, most notorious of all, the hammerhead stall. It was a beautiful day. Blue skies, sunshine and not a breeze, nor a cloud, to be found. A perfect day to fly, and hopefully not a perfect day to die! This adventure was testing the limits of my favorite motto: I'll try anything once, twice if I like it and I don't kill myself. This adventure was truly fitting for that.

We met up at a small regional airport just outside of Temecula. He led me to a sleek looking number and helped me climb aboard. Once inside, he handed me a pair of goggles, and a leather aviator's hat, purely for effect. If we were to hit the ground, the hat would be wearing me. The engine started and my excitement grew. Or was it my nervousness? It was hard to differentiate between the two. Maybe it was a perfect mixture of both. I was seated directly behind Peter. Once the safety checklist was performed, we taxied to the end of the runway, made a quick turn, and began to pick up speed, as the propellers kicked into gear. A few hundred yards later we were airborne.

The flight began with a few final safety tips, namely pointing out the location of a backup steering tiller, which happened to be between my legs. There was also a short lesson on how the back-up throttle worked, which is always a hope that it would not become necessary. Moments later I heard the words, "you are in control" and he handed the steering tiller over to me. But I could see a cautious hand steady on the main tiller in front of me. Shortly after taking control again, he took the plane into a sharp sweeping horizontal curve and the excitement overtook the nervousness. As the plane straightened out, I thought to myself that it was a great ride. The next thing I knew we were in a loop-the-loop, where the plane makes three consecutive vertical circles, thus pinning my body into the seat. Almost immediately following the conclusion of that stunt, the plane flipped upside down in a barrel roll set.

The only problem was that coming out of the third roll, I did not have control of my legs. Once we flipped over for the last time, my leg came down on the steering tiller. He promptly grabbed on with both hands, and gave me an opportunity to straighten out my legs, which at this point were fully spasming. Just as soon as everything was back in order, he performed the cout-de-gras. The plane picked up speed and we were headed directly towards the heavens, in what was known as a hammerhead stall. The plane strained to keep going upward, but abruptly the engine stopped. Although it was nice and quiet, I couldn't help but be concerned about the lack of an engine. The plane fell off to the right side, and amidst the deep dive, I heard the comforting sound of an engine. I was asked if I wanted to do a few more tricks, but I politely declined. I was done for the day.

He explained the reason for the engine failing to be the inability of the engine to pump gas and keep the combustion going. Sounds simple, but in the moment frayed every single nerve in my body.

FREE FALLING – PART 3

We pulled off the freeway just outside of Perris, California and proceeded down the gravel driveway 100 yards, to a freestanding small trailer. A lean, casually dressed man and came up and quickly introduced himself as Joe Jennings. Just as soon as we were introduced, he was saying, "I'll be right back" and abruptly ran off to join five other individuals loading necessities into the waiting plane. As my friend, Steve, and I unloaded our chairs from the car, we watched the plane taxi down the runway and take off. Almost as soon as we had finished gathering our equipment, the plane was landing, and Joe met back up with us in the makeshift office. Piled up against the wall, and stacked four rows/columns deep were numerous boxes, which he explained were filled with 5 x 8 logbooks, that recorded thousands of his prior jumps.

Steve had explained, on the ride to the airfield, that Joe was known as a "go-to" guy in Hollywood if you needed something, anything, related to parachuting. He had worked as a stunt double on numerous movies, including the famous scene with Harrison Ford throwing bad guys out of the back of "Air Force One." "Get off my plane!", I'm sure you're saying in your head right now.

After filling out the requisite liability paperwork, we were soon gearing up in the cliché, neon-colored jumpsuits, leather helmet and aviator goggles. Joe gave us a very brief outline of what to expect. We transferred from our earthbound wheelchairs, into the side of a cargo plane, with the propellers gently spinning. What a false sense of calm those propellers were. Soon we were taxiing down the runway and lifting off the familiar, calming terra firma. We sat on the floor of the plane, and as it climbed in altitude, I climbed in anxious anticipation; a direct positive correlation. I could see the earth getting farther and farther away, through the modified, rollup, acrylic door. Soon the instructors, that we were soon to attach ourselves to, started to stir, and encouraged us to inch closer to the slowly-opening rollup door. I watched as a woman with a VHS camera climbed out the door, along the side of the plane, to a seemingly microscopic, and precarious, spot on top of the wing strut. This same VHS tape would, sometime later, get me in trouble with my wife, who found the incriminating evidence while I was away on a work trip.

Steve was the first one scheduled to jump. More realistically it was going to be a skid and slide, out of the plane. At least I would get to watch him first. Being concerned with last-minute safety details, all I saw was him exiting the plane. Suddenly, it was my turn. My adrenaline level shot off the charts as we edged toward the door opening. Was it too late to turn around? Joe sat behind me and clipped to the harness on my back. Next came a detail that I "missed" in the pre-flight instruction. I was to scoot through the door opening and literally hang, suspended from his harness. The "1-2-3" count seemed to take an eternity before being guided out. But before we know it, I was freefalling through the atmosphere, of course with my new friend Joe. What a rush it was! Whatever anxiety I was feeling soon gave way to being fully in the moment. Before too long, I felt a tap on my shoulder and heard him say "it's almost time to pull the cord". I had all but forgotten to check my altimeter telling me when to slow the dissent. I anxiously fumbled for the ripcord, without success, until a steadying hand guided me to location and assisted me in pulling.

Thankfully, the shoot gently deployed and brought us to a screeching halt, providing the sensation of being in reverse, back towards the sky. At this point Joe took over and worked the thermals and flow gently towards the dots that represented our wheelchairs, barely even visible. Soon came the most critical part: landing. Too slow and we risked the possibility of getting swept away from our target. Too fast and I might end up a couple feet shorter. But he proved his expertise almost effortlessly, and gently landed beside my chair, with Steve waiting nearby. We shared in each other's excitement and recounted the process. Just as soon as we had arrived, we were loading back in the car with our souvenir photos and videotape. We watched as another car pulled in the parking lot, four individuals climbing out, anticipating their turn at defying gravity. I couldn't help but feel excitement for them, knowing what lie ahead.

All of these activities might seem out of reach for those who are otherwise afflicted. But each was an indescribable thrill of a lifetime and lead me to friends, connections and other experiences that I would never have had. Always ask about accommodations – most are more than happy to help in your participation or will recommend someone they know who can.

CHAPTER 7

30ᵀᴴ BIRTHDAY CROSSOVER

I was casually sitting in Earl's living room in Santa Cruz, with the seminal 30th birthday rapidly approaching. Instead of stressing over this societally-imposed milestone, I decided it was a good excuse for an adventure on par with 30 years of life. To boot, I was up for going literally anywhere in the world. Having been going nonstop for the last 3 years, and then some, I had forgotten to take a break, and gone without a vacation. Work, starting a business and swim training had taken the driver's seat – a social life was in the trunk. It was time.

I had been working full time at a van conversion company assisting physically challenged individuals in determining the necessary equipment to adapt their vehicle and get them mobile, driving. In addition, Charlie and I had started a business aptly named "Chair – a – Van", renting wheelchair accessible vans and providing transportation in the San Francisco Bay Area and throughout California. In our years of traveling for business, pleasure and various sporting activities we would often want to do trip adjacent travel to see other places around the U.S. The biggest obstacle was often lack of accessible transportation at the destinations. Unable to transfer into a car, because it hadn't yet been properly equipped, we decided to take matters into our own hands. For us, and others similarly situated this was important work.

During this time period swim training in preparation for the '88 Seoul Paralympics had ramped up to two times per day, 6 am. and 7 pm, 5 to 6 days a week. A secret: it was almost always 6 days. After finishing the morning swim workout, it was off to work by 9 am at the latest, to put in a full day. I would then grab a quick dinner and head to the evening "Water Wheels" swim team workout. In addition, we were attending various swim meets across the U.S. and internationally. My schedule was bananas and looking back I'm not sure where that energy came from.

This hectic schedule had been going continuously for the past two years, or so. I lost count. To put it in a nutshell I was burnt out, as evidenced by a recent car collision on the freeway after briefly nodding off. In the process of the accident, I scraped with center guard rail. Somehow, the state of California was able to determine that this relatively minor scrape on the well-worn guard rail was worth $666. Was that a coincidence, or prophetic? Either way, it was cause for pause. Maybe also some re-evaluation, but only after quality R&R.

It was going to be a chance for a solo trip, which I value highly, even crave. So, we brought out the World Atlas and lay it on the coffee table. The first thought was to visit and swim with the big turtles of the Galápagos Islands and raft the Amazon rainforest. After some research, I decided that entailed too much travel time and involved too many transfers on and off puddle jumper planes and boats. Airplane transfers are anything but simple in a chair. Ask my frequent travel companions, my family. The second possibility was to sail around the Greek Islands, snorkeling, scuba diving, fishing, soaking up sun, eating, drinking, and having some general fun. Unfortunately, these two options required about a day's worth of travel time each direction. We looked for something a little bit closer.

In keeping with the island theme, I thought it might be nice to head down to the Tahitian islands and spend a little time on the beach. And while in the neighborhood thought it might be nice to head down under to Australia to catch up with a few friends made through swimming. The final plan was to go to the secluded Island of Morea for a week and unplug from society and try to regain some perspective. This was to be followed by a week on the party island of Bora Bora to start the 30th birthday celebration. And then for a unique twist, I would get on a flight to Australia, crossing the international date line at approximately midnight on the day before my 30th birthday, thus jumping ahead one day. In essence missing my 30th birthday. There was no special reason to do the dateline birthday crossover other than it seemed like a cool thing to do and that it would make a good life story.

More on that later.

The flight from S.F. to Tahiti International Airport was fairly uneventful. Always a welcome surprise. The much smaller 4 seat prop plane flight to the island of Morea reminded me of a 70s show, 'Fantasy Island', as we circled over the lush island paradise surrounded by white sand beaches. Suddenly, a single landing strip appears over the top of the palm trees. The hotel transport was waiting at the single hanger airport, and we took the Jeep ride on dirt roads to my bungalow hideaway for the next week. This was going to be an opportunity to catch up on my reading in the shade of a palm tree with a gentle tropical breeze blowing and an umbrella drink in hand. Or so the vision in my mind went. The front porch of the cabin faced the ocean providing spectacular sunsets. The only time interacting with anyone would be by choice, or when going for a meal at the common dining area. Other than that, I slept, read, had a few Tahini Beers and gazed at the water and fantasized about a life spent traveling the islands. It was just what Dr. Feelgood ordered.

One day, while on a push down a path lined with gorgeous bougainvillea, camellias and other beautiful flora indigenous to the region, I made the acquaintance of an elderly local resident. He loaned me his binoculars to watch the birds and a pod of humpback whales as they breached, playing and feeding their young on their journey south for their annual breeding. This experience was like a living page from National Geographic. This was exactly the decompression, the reset that I needed. It was a true reconnection with nature. After a week, the batteries were fully recharged, and it was time to have a little fun Tahiti style. So, I took the puddle jumper from tiny and quiet

Morea to the more upbeat island of Bora Bora. It was the laidback party island for the rich and the beautiful. It brought to mind a long-held fantasy of island hopping with Jimmy Buffett playing in the background, or a private show. Either would be fine by me.

The island of Bora Bora is relatively small, with approximately 7,000 full time residents in a total of 10 square miles. All was surrounded by motus with a dirt road encircling the dormant volcano of Mt. Otematu. For reference, I live in a medium-sized college town now and the student attendance alone far surpasses the full-time residency of the island. The physical size of our town is at least twice that. This is exactly why I love to travel; the juxtaposition and cultural learning opportunities.

While planning for the trip, in an effort to keep costs down, I called the Tahiti Department of Tourism and inquired about the possibility of camping while on the islands. I heard a brief laugh on the other end of the phone and the voice said, "We don't have camping in Tahiti". So, I ended up booking a room at the Maheata Hotel, which came out to $110 per night. That will get you a nice hotel room even with today's currency rates. So back in 1987, you can imagine my hesitancy and questioning at that price tag. But without any options I just had to suck it up.

One upside to vacationing in warm weather locations is that luggage is much lighter and easier to handle. This is paramount to maneuvering for a more positive experience, and hotel accommodations.

Arriving at the hotel, I had reconciled myself to the fact that I was going to be working to pay off this bill upon my return to the states, and checked in. I proceeded to make my way to find my "accessible room", only to be met by an 8-inch threshold to enter the room. Managing to pop the front wheels of my chair up and on the room floor and literally pulling myself into the room, I wondered how many times I would perform this until I decided I wouldn't do it anymore. The room itself was nice with tropically themed décor with a slowly oscillating palm leaf fan creating a gentle breeze. As I moved about the room checking out the facilities, I discovered that the doorway to the bathroom was about 3 inches too narrow for me to enter without a repeat performance of the front door scene. It would require a transfer from the wheelchair to a chair placed inside the door, and then to the toilet, or shower tub. So now this relatively expensive accessible hotel room was officially indeed not accessible at all and still just as expensive. To say the least, I was bummed out, bordering on intensely irritated. Prior to leaving home, I had called the hotel confirming the accessibility of the room. I was assured that it was wheelchair accessible. When I talked to the hotel manager, I explained the situation and that I had been assured accessibility. Of course, they had no record of the call and proved inflexible to negotiating a deal, or maybe just truly unable. So, I cogitated on my next steps and decided that heading to town and having a beer was the right thing to do.

On the way down the road toward town, I was rolling past a quaint village with a cluster of houses and family businesses when I noticed out of the corner of my eye a small sign with the word "camping" painted on it. Simple yet effective. They had my attention. I approached an elderly, well-tanned shirtless man working in the yard, and he turned out to be the property owner. Was my luck turning around? I asked him what the deal was with the camping sign and recounted the conversation with the Tourism Department. He informed me that the hotels on the island had pressured the government to include that spiel when inquiring minds came along, citing the weakened economy and potential effect on their bottom line.

The magic words I heard next, "A spot on the beach is five dollars per night".

I looked at the area to which he was pointing and saw a white sand beach, where the crystal blue water gently lapped on the shore. He could see obvious disappointment on my face. I responded, "that's too bad because I was told there wasn't camping and didn't bring a tent or sleeping bag". He came back with, "you don't need a tent because of the mellow tropical nights," and mentioned that if I had wanted, he could rent out a tent for five dollars a night. He generously threw in a sleeping bag for another five, if I was interested. It was a done deal.

Newly energized from the discovery, I continued into town and headed to the bar to enjoy a couple beers. On the way back to the hotel, I checked in at the "campground" and made arrangements for a spot on the beach for the following day. Then I headed to the hotel desk to promptly adjust my reservation from there on out. Fifteen minutes later, I was checked out of the "accessible" room, and into the new beachfront address for the remainder of my stay on the island. The too expensive hotel room had just gotten $100 cheaper, and the evening meal suddenly tasted a lot better. The following morning, I took the time to get the lay of the land, simply the sand and the waves, and my "room". It was a burnt orange tent on the beach. All I had to do was cross approximately 10 feet of white sand and I was at the clearest blue water I had ever seen. During the check-in process, I met the owner's son and we immediately hit it off. His name was Oscar, and he was the maintenance person for the business. That night while sitting in the door of my tent, watching the sunset over the islands with the sound of perfect tunes floating through the air from a local building, I saw Oscar out of the corner of my eye, approaching with a glass in each hand. In the glass was a tropical punch concoction with plenty of rum. Happy hour had begun. Following the cocktails, he disappeared and returned with a dinner consisting of a fresh salad and the fresh caught mahi-mahi, that he had found earlier that day. I recalled having seen him earlier in the day with a large fish slung over his shoulder. I was fortunate enough that he chose to share that catch with me. That night I fell asleep to the sound of gentle waves as they reached the shore. My dreams that night were merely fantasies of what it would be like to just sail from island to island on nobody's schedule but my own.

The next morning, I slowly woke to the sound of my name being called from outside the tent flap. It was Oscar with a hot cup of freshly ground coffee and a plate of freshly sliced fruit and croissant. We exchanged pleasantries and shared a slice of the morning, while the sun gradually warmed the sand. He informed me that the Tahitian government frowned upon camping, like I was doing, so as not to take business away from the local resorts and hotels. After finishing the coffee, he disappeared yet again, only to reemerge with a second cup of coffee and a bowl of fresh fruit and a freshly baked scone. If he wasn't careful, he was going to end up being my new best friend. What a great start to the day.

After breakfast I scooted across the sand with a mask and snorkel that I had borrowed from Oscar. With the gear on, I slipped into the 80 degree water, for a morning swim and to observe the sea life that existed an arm's length away from my tent. How was any of this even possible? It was late morning when I headed into town to explore on land and find some lunch. As I was leaving the campground, I met another young American, named Nick, from New York. After brief introductions, we headed into town together. After lunch and a couple beers at Bloody Mary's, we decided to hitchhike on the way back to the campground. It was only a couple of miles along the main dirt road but for some reason we decided hitchhiking was the best option. I threw my thumb in the air, and almost immediately a black Jeep pulled over just down the road. I thought to myself that hitchhiking in Tahiti is pretty easy. I should have reserved my judgment.

However, as we approached the Jeep, the two occupants stumbled out of the vehicle, along with a few beer cans and proceeded to the side of the road to relieve themselves. At this point, I had decided to slow my roll so as not to startle them. The last thing I wanted was to have them turn their hoses on me. I asked the driver if he could give us a ride to the campground and he neutrally agreed. So, I climbed into the front passenger seat and put the frame of my chair on my lap while Nick and the other passenger got in the back. As we cruised down the road, I asked the driver "what kind of work you do on Bora Bora for a living"? "I'm an outrigger canoe tour operator". *Ding ding*. The sound of a bell chimed loudly in my head, as another wild idea took up residence in my brain. You can sense a theme here. I explained the background story of my trip, and that tomorrow was the last day I was spending on the island. I would be catching a flight mid-evening, heading to Sydney, Australia. I wanted to end with a highlight.

"I was hoping to go on an outrigger canoe tour of the islands before leaving," I blurted out. He replied that he would love to take me for a tour, but he had a really important meeting in the morning.

And playing the part of the somewhat typical, arrogant American, I sarcastically implored, "what's so important that you can't take me for a tour around the islands"? He explained that he had a very important meeting in the morning with the Minister of Tourism, to discuss possible solutions to a recent downturn in the tourism industry. *Ding ding*. Off goes another bell in my mind.

"How cool would the minister think you were if you not only brought an American tourist, but one in a wheelchair to discuss the state of the tourism industry?"

I did have a knack for nabbing an invite.

This time, I could see the wheels turning in his head. Soon we had made arrangements for a 9 AM pickup on my porch; the beach in front of my tent. That night's dinner was more fresh fish in a bowl with rice and fresh vegetables. I think today it is popularly known as a poke bowl. And before I knew it, I was relaxing, dozing off, to the sounds of gentle water and light breezes flowing through the palm trees, cogitating the next day's potential adventures. It was going to be exciting, to say the least.

The next morning, I woke up to fresh coffee and fruit and another morning dip in the surreal blue water. Truly indescribable. As I prepared for my date with the Minister, the 9 o'clock hour rolled around quicker than anticipated. No canoe. 9:15 came and went, still no canoe. I was starting to think that Rusty had likely continued on with his night of drinking, and was sleeping it off, or that bringing me along was going to be an unnecessary hassle. All of these were reasonable, fair points. Suddenly, in the distance, the sound of a small outboard motor could be heard. Around the corner came a six person outrigger canoe, slowly approaching the beach. He softly glided the front end into the sand. Before I could blink, he had taken out the middle seat and put my wheelchair in its place. I less than laboriously climbed in, and we were off to the island of Raiatea. We were greeted on the private government island by the minister of tourism and several servants. We were escorted into the dining room and provided with a somewhat formal lunch, which included what was referred to as a "rich mans" salad. The main ingredient was the heart of a local palm tree, somewhat akin to an artichoke heart. The reason for the name is that the palm tree will have given its life to provide this delicacy for us.

After lunch we retreated to a cabana room, where we were offered seating in large, luxurious cushioned lounge chairs. We were brought coffee and cigars, followed up by a punch cocktail. This proved to be the business part of the day. The minister of tourism started in with facts and figures about the state of the tourist economy and recent declines. He turned to me, asking my opinion of what Tahiti had to offer from a tourist's perspective, and how to increase the tourist numbers. I provided him with a countenance of my wonderful experiences of the islands up to that point. It couldn't all be blowing smoke. I did also provide an in-depth suggestion that I thought would increase tourism numbers.

"The cost of everything is unjustifiably expensive."

I followed that statement up by explaining the concept of the "meter drop". Of course, you always get people with money to come to Tahiti for a getaway. However, it is not those swimming in cash that sustain the businesses, it is their "regular" counterparts. In other words, instead of relying on the "home run", you support the economy by hitting a larger number of "singles" and "doubles". Somehow, he seemed amazed at this logic and promised to incorporate it into his plans. We then headed outside for a ceremonial planting of several palm trees, a gesture in remembrance of the ones that were part of lunch.

By the time we had concluded our chat it was mid-afternoon, and my flight was scheduled for 7 o'clock that evening, which was quickly approaching. We decided to head back to Bora Bora. We pulled away from Raiatea in the canoe. Once out of the site of the minister, my guide pulled out what looked to be a hand-rolled cigarette. It quickly became apparent that he was offering for me to indulge in some local harmless plant. So as not to seem ungrateful, I "reluctantly" agreed to partake. It wasn't reluctance at all. Then we began what seemed to be a fantasy tour of the islands, complete with the sun setting through the palm trees. At this point, I was truly in a National Geographic commercial. After indulging a few more times, we glided through the water, past several other islands in the chain. I suddenly realized the setting sun in the background meant that it was almost 6 o'clock. We still needed to get back to Bora Bora pack up my stuff and head the airport. So, we put the canoe "in gear" and headed towards home.

Part of the plan this trip for that was hatched on the couch several months prior was to leave Tahiti the night before my birthday, flying to Sydney. Coincidently I would be crossing the international date line at midnight. That would catapult me forward a whole day, thus in essence "skipping" my 30th birthday. I didn't plan this because I was bothered by the milestone, but more because it seemed like a cool idea and was feasible to plan. The other big concept behind the plan was to have yin and yang. A juxtaposition on this milestone birthday, to go from laying on the beach, and tropical climates, to snow skiing, within a matter of hours. It seemed like an appropriate representation of my life as it had played out up to now. Hopefully, balance and contrast would stay put as a theme in my life.

Unfortunately, that entire day leading up to my flight proved too frenzied, followed by imbibing, persuading us to take in the islands in more laid-back fashion. More life symbolism for me. In any event I missed my flight. I rebooked on the 11 o'clock flight and essentially saw about seven hours of my 30th birthday, instead of zero. More apt allegory there. Oh well, the best laid plans as they say…

I made it to Australia without further theatrics. But I did find some good trouble to get into upon arrival and brief exploration. First, a tad bit of background.

Back home in California, I had tried adaptive cross-country snow-skiing, which was basically sledding with minimal control. I liked it enough to try and find something similar down under. Those that I came in contact with while in Australia had come up with a new device, which included a molded plastic seat mounted on an early version of the snowboard, called a Swingbo. My inaugural attempt on this new invention, I was able to turn with ease under total control. This made for a good, relatively adventurous portion of the trip. The inventors were eager to tap into the U.S. market, and before leaving I had agreed to do some research with plans of becoming the U.S. distributor, or ambassador. Upon returning stateside, one of the first steps was to inquire about insurance for this new business. I had learned the hard way from a previous business venture that procuring insurance for an adaptive equipment business was difficult. The several meetings with insurance reps went something like this. "Let me get this straight, you want to take someone with a physical disability, strap them on a ski machine and send them down a hill covered with snow and ice?" I replied "Yes". After 6 rejections, including specialty insurers Lloyds of London, their overall resounding answer was "NO!".

I guess they just weren't quite ready.

As for the rest of the Australian portion of the trip goes, I will keep that between myself and those who actively participated. After all, this is just a highlight reel, not a play-by-play.

CHAPTER 8

VOLGELSANG

The Yosemite Valley floor was spectacular, but looking up at the surrounding mountains and monoliths, I began to realize there was so much more. Conversations with experienced rock climbers left me wanting to experience all the High Sierras had to offer. I discussed an idea with a longtime friend, who was a strong hiker and climber. The idea revolved around the potential of rigging up a harness that would allow him to lead and me to follow. Meaning I would be tethered to him, and another attachment to my chair frame. We would be working our way into the clouds and ultimately to high country this way. He was willing to take on the challenge, so we began to plan the intricacies of this excursion. It was going to take a lot of detail, and variables to cooperate with us. I wanted the full experience of climbing, allowing me to do as much work as possible, which is tricky. Over the course of one winter in the mid '90's, we had developed specialized rigging; a harness that would go over his shoulders and attach to the front of my chair, that with coordinated effort would enable us to attempt to climb the steep terrain. We determined an appropriate route out of Tuolumne Meadows, along the creek, and finally up to the high country known as Vogelsang.

Unfortunately, a couple months prior to the planned departure, John experienced a severe fall, which caused a debilitating back injury, eliminating any possibility of him providing his Sherpa-like assistance services. Needless to say, all of our planning and hard work was for naught; this trip was tabled, indefinitely. The stars that we needed to align, simply didn't.

I was on a separate solo camping excursion to Tuolumne Meadows sometime after this "grounded flight", located in the more remote eastern side of Yosemite, when I noticed mules and a stable. This sight gave me yet another idea. This beautiful area off of Highway 140 and Tioga Pass was often less traveled. This was due to the late snowpack on Tioga Road, which causes road closure through May and into June. Less traveled doesn't always equal bad. I went in for a closer look and struck up a conversation with a stable hand. He explained that the mules were there to take supplies up to the high sierra camps, which provided luxury camping for the less adventurous. I explained my desire to experience the high country, and how it was put on hold with my friends back injury. As we talked, the idea took shape, and I inquired about the possibility of hitching a ride to the high country, for a week of camping. And I was met with a very matter-of-fact, "Sure. We'll put you on one mule and your chair and equipment on another. In fact, we happen to have a cancellation, and availability for tomorrow". Although tempted, I was unprepared to make the proposed trip on a day's notice. But before I left the stables, I had made a commitment to return.

Two weeks later, I was mounting a mule and on my way to the high country. As stable hands packed my gear on one mule, it was all-hands-on-deck in an attempt to figure out a way to get me on top of the other mule. We would put two pair hands on one side of the mule to lift and push, with someone on the other side to catch just in case I was boosted too forcibly. After much pulling and tugging, I was atop the mule.

The trail out of Tuolumne Meadows followed the river and wound through beautiful pastoral splendor, with a carpet of California wildflowers blooming all around. Completing the picture, were remnants of the spring melt, as evidenced by the seasonal lakes. The vast meadow slowly narrowed into a trail, which we followed as we climbed steadily uphill, for the next three plus hours. Following Murphy Creek, we ascended into the high country. The trail was steep and narrow. The mules thankfully were surefooted as advertised, at times plodding and lumbering on a trail that, in certain devilish spots, was only 8 inches wide. They did so with a quiet confidence. This did wonders to assuage my extremely raw nerves. After a full day of climbing, we were suddenly at 11,000 feet. Just as soon as we arrived at the edge of the high Sierra camp up popped a summer shower.

There lie Vogelsang. I had finally made it.

CHAPTER 9

ROCK N' ROLL YOSEMITE

It was a particularly rainy winter for California. In fact, that year and the year prior had seen unmatched flooding, and sheer volume of water. Wish we could have those times back, instead of the current unending drought. It was late January, and the setting was once again Earl's living room, where we were complaining about that rainy weather. We were thumbing through a travel magazine, dreaming of potential getaways from this deluge downfall. There was an article in VIA magazine about Yosemite and the conversation then drifted to Yosemite National Park. My oft travel partner then promptly recounted his numerous experiences travelling there. I had yet to experience it's wonder. All of this talk was increasing my desire to go to this beautiful national treasure, which was in our backyard, a mere 4 hours away.

One of the good things about an above average amount of rainfall in the Northern California's Central Valley is the massive snowpack it builds in the Sierra mountains. This, in turn, feeds the area during the arid summers. This same snowpack also feeds the Merced River, as it winds through Yosemite Valley and supplies water for the park's spectacular waterfalls. We decided that an early spring journey to the park would be in order. While researching the trip over the next two months, we looked at the camping options as well as the many exploration opportunities. While thumbing through a brochure put out by the National Parks, I noticed a 20-mile trail around the valley floor, which was designated as accessible bike trail. Since the distance was too far to push and I was becoming an avid hand-cyclist, we decided to include bikes on the trip just in case the opportunity arose. Always prepared or pretending to be.

We met in Groveland, a small mountain town about an hour outside Yosemite in early May. The plan was to caravan toward our campsite on the valley floor. Stopping at the park entrance we were talking to a park ranger about various programs offered in the park and the associated entry fee, charged by the federal government. One of the rangers informed us about the "Golden Access" pass, which provided free national park entrance to all individuals with qualifying disabilities. This was a good thing because the $20 entry fee was unaccounted for in our shoestring budget. Another reason to ask or get people talking as often as possible.

Our campsite was in an area known as the Lower Pines, which provided water and a relatively flat and accessible surrounding area. Immediately upon arrival at our spot, we decided to skip unpacking and to jump on our bikes for a reconnaissance mission to check out the neighborhood. We spent the rest of the daylight hours checking out the immediate area and parts of the accessible bike trail, hoping to add that to tomorrow's agenda. We pulled back into the campsite just as the sun was setting, being filtered through the mist generated by Bridal Veil Falls. This required us to set up camp in the dark. Not ideal in any circumstance. Over a late-evening dinner around the campfire, we discussed the next day's adventures and eventually drifted off to sleep. I decided to try the full camping experience and set up my bed on the ground, on a mat of pine needles, while Earl decided on the comfort of his VW Vanagon. Needless to say, I was worse for the wear the next day. I experienced unwelcome soreness caused by the hard ground, several ill-located rocks and dagger-like pinecones, previously veiled by the dark. I understood how the princess from the Princess and the Pea story, that I used to read to my daughter, felt.

The soreness quickly dissipated as we awoke to the spectacular site of the sunrise reflecting and refracting off the granite monolith of Half Dome, magnificently filtering through the trees. To round out the intense but amazing sensory experience, Yosemite Falls was thundering in the background. All 5 senses, plus some, were definitely fully engaged. We anxiously inhaled our breakfast and mounted our bikes for the morning's adventure to the east end of the valley. Included on the map: Happy Isles, Mirror Lake and Half Dome. Never having cycled around the valley, I was unsure of the accuracy of the route in comparison to the brochure, and what exactly they considered accessible. Everywhere seems to have a different definition. Throughout the years, I learned that lesson the hard way on other adventures. The path out of the campsite to the morning destinations was a combination of sidewalks, roads and bike trails. All of these were wheelchair accessible and situated on roads with relatively no traffic. Another lesson I learned from previous experiences was to go before Memorial Day or after Labor Day, to avoid an onslaught of tourists. Given the distance we had to cover and time limitations, bikes proved to be the most excellent option. We toured the east end of the valley that morning, making sure to take time and soak in the beauty and majesty around every corner. The ultimate highlight of the morning was the awe-inspiring granite monolith of Half Dome. We strained our necks to take in the enormity of this sheer edifice, being forced to look straight up to take it all in. A straight shot to the top; ground level to 7000 feet.

We briefly stopped back at camp for a quick and small lunch, before heading out for our afternoon adventures. The afternoon found us on a longer ride, 15 miles or so, around the west end of the valley. This route took us through Yosemite Village, past Yosemite Falls, El Capitan and Bridal Veil Falls. As we biked around the valley floor, it seemed like around every corner there were even more spectacular sites to behold. We had to take care on this segment, as parts of the bike trail were on active roadways. Because others navigating the narrow roadways in 2-ton vehicles were also taking in the same majestic sights, it created a potentially dangerous situation for those of us on bikes. However, you can correctly assume, since I am writing this, that we made it out alive. Not without a few close calls. The day's exercise in the mountain air, coupled with the white noise of Yosemite Falls in the background, helped sleep to come easy that night.

The next morning proved even more difficult to get my aching body out of bed than the day prior. With only half of a day left to explore, we decided to take the newly constructed accessible path to lower Yosemite Falls. Although, the path to the falls proved difficult, with a couple turns too sharp for the elongated hand cycles. If you have never operated one, the turning radius and steering on a hand cycle doesn't happen on a dime. The most difficult part of this portion was to explain to the other park visitors what we were riding. We received a few negative comments complaining about riding bikes on the path. Since our time left was limited, we tried to brush them off as quickly as possible.

As the path neared the falls, the roar came to a crescendo. We found ourselves suddenly on a small bridge with the base of the thundering Yosemite falls, which was generating a thick mist. The falls were merely an arm's length away. My hat was nearly offered to the river god, from the power that the falls generated, saved by a nearby tourist with quick reflexes. Similar scenes to the one with my hat, played in a seemingly endless loop for our duration of the trek, with any and all visitors. I felt like Bill Murray in the movie Groundhog's Day.

Upon arriving back at the camp, we decided that, since we had traveled this far, and we were having the experience of a lifetime, that we might as well stay another day. The magic that is Yosemite, had taken over the decision-making process. We also made a promise that we would be back, like the Terminator.

The awesomeness that Yosemite had to offer, combined with ease of access that the handcycle provided, gave rise to an idea. How can we possibly open up the extraordinary exploration opportunity we had just experienced, in the future to others with various physical challenges? Upon returning home, we sprung into action to make this plan a reality. My life is a continuous loop of a select few themes. This is one of them.

To get going on the actual planning for this dream event, the City of Sacramento, Access Leisure program was contacted. We set up an appointment to meet and discuss the experience, and potential of combining forces to offer said experience to a larger group. The City currently offered a local handcycling program, which introduced the sport to the interested individuals and provided supported rides, limited to the area. The idea of a camping trip to Yosemite seemed to be a natural extension of the local program. In the back of our minds, questions came up: was it feasible and was it actionable? Those were the two practical, logistical, large-scale questions, and were accompanied by at least 100 more hair-splitters.

As we gathered around the conference table, I recounted my personal recent handcycling adventure. I talked about being among surrounding natural wonders, and the ease with which I navigated, due to the handcycle. However,

I wondered about the accessibility required to organize a trip scaled for a larger group. I was fully expecting to have this somewhat aggressive idea rejected. But the forward-thinking Supervisor, Annie, simply said, "Sounds good. You put it together and we'll make it happen". Additionally, she offered any support and input she could provide. Annie's endorsement, along with Earl's efforts, his High Sierra experience, and high energy that he always had stored for a rainy day, created a dream team that put the plan into motion, and intensely.

Over the next 6 months, we made two planning trips in the spring, and one in fall, for a total of three scouting trips to the park. The purpose of these trips was to develop the foundation of the trip, including critical details of housing, food, and the route. The main idea was to provide a challenging "naturalized" camping experience in this national backyard jewel, while accommodating for a variety of unique physical challenges. The final version of the route was ultimately similar to my very first experience, with a few modifications and adaptations. On one of these previous planning trips that had been made to the park, a meeting was set with the park rangers to clarify why the use of handcycles were necessary for our mobility. They appreciated the heads up and indicated that the handcycles would be acceptable as adaptive equipment to get to the falls. There were so many details and plans that had to be carefully laid, so that when half inevitably fell through, we still had a solid foundation and could execute this excursion.

The biggest planning challenge was housing, as there were three limiting factors. In order to accommodate the largest number of participants, we had to accommodate for campsite accessibility, ability to experience as much of the natural surroundings as possible and keeping cost reasonable. Three things about housing; needed to accommodate as many as possible for financial purposes, needed to be physically accessible, needed to incorporate education, along with campfires and s'mores. We quickly realized that some people would have difficulty camping on the ground, and others would not be able to afford the price of the various housing options within the park. The workaround for this particular issue came in the Housekeeping Camp. Formerly used to house workers in the Valley, these three-sided units were minimally equipped, with cement flooring, a tarp roof and a curtain door. Inside the cabins there were simply one double bed, two bunk beds and a 110 V outlet. Each little gathering of cabins had a faucet that provided fresh water, and a fire pit to gather around – popular activities included singing and roasting marshmallows for s'mores. This was the balance we were looking for.

We also put in a request to internationally-renowned Mark Wellman to join and provide his expertise. To me, Mark was simply a good buddy. He was a former park ranger and the first paraplegic to climb half-dome and El Capitan, after sustaining a severe injury to his back, which found him on the other side as paraplegic.

Mark was able to arrange a separate meeting with park rangers and the High Sierra Climbing school, to incorporate an additional facet of this trip; a once in a lifetime experience climbing the actual granite walls of Yosemite. He was also the owner of NoLimitsTahoe.com, which has since branched and expanded well beyond my pay grade. The website is where you could read more about his story and experiences and get in contact about motivational speaking engagements.

We successfully turned this vision into a reality, and a regular trip for a not-so-regular group of humans.

Some of the fondest memories for all were had in that valley, near those waterfalls, and in those pesky tents. The group learned a lot, and had tons of fun as well. A win-win. A long-running success.

EPILOGUE

BEHIND THE SCENES, AND A POST-RICKY WORLD

What you read throughout the course of this story is just a brief glimpse into one man's journey, post-paralysis and diagnosis. From that day forward, every single day was an uphill battle, but one that he was willing to endure, find the beauty in, and thrive as a result.

So much was left out of this story; his experiences with other sports endeavors, coaching, parenting and a homelife in general, other notable career experiences and what lead him to them, and details behind the scenes of what we do not see as typically-abled people. While he is humble enough to not tell you every detail, I will share a bit more of what made him… him.

He was a great athlete, plagued by further injuries as he aged – handcycling, wheelchair rugby, tennis in addition to his swimming success, in his younger years. With handcycling, he was known in town (and the surrounding towns) for his daily rides. He was planning and ready to execute a cross-country cycle trip until a doctor's exam left him with the realization that he was doing permanent damage to his shoulders if he continued. Handcycling forced him to step back and take on a new role, shifting his perspective after that. Wheelchair rugby was his true sports love, if you ask me. He lived for the thrill. He was a founding member of the west coast branch of the wheelchair rugby association (USQRA), determined to expand and get more quads involved in the sport. A teacher of mine growing up bonded with him over his "gnarly badassery" for his enthusiastic participation in quad rugby. Of course, rugby, especially wheelchair rugby, takes a toll. That lifestyle could not be sustained forever. Tennis was a feat, and something he found himself not having too much time for after the early nineties, but he was truly an ace. Pun intended. Swimming was a fewer and farther between recreational activity, but one that he enjoyed at home, especially in the triple digit summers.

From there, coaching was a natural transition, and almost seemed like a role he was meant to be in from the start. Many who know him the best joke that he missed his calling as a life coach. He just knew so much about so many things. It was uncanny really. But I am of the strong opinion that he served his peers, his community, his ecosphere very well as a coach, both in wheelchair rugby and wheelchair softball. He modeled that coaching goes far beyond game strategies, training and winning. It was about connections and applications. Making human connections, forming relationships from there and also taking what you learn on the court or the field, and applying it in the world. He taught me how to be an athlete, and now that I am an adult, how to be a coach but still take care of my body and pursue appropriate athletic endeavors.

Another missing part of the story was his homelife. As the youngest sibling, he had four amazing nieces. Two from each sibling. But his life was not on anyone else's timeline or lived by anyone else's expectations. There was no hurry, for anything. He unexpectedly met a wonderful woman, a few years his senior, and they decided that if they wanted to try to have a baby they should do so, sooner rather than later. Both had potential limitations working against them. Though society STILL often frowns upon kids before marriage, they got lucky pretty quickly. The pair of them were blessed with a hell-raising, smart-mouthed daughter shortly after they decided to try for a child. She was a handful and proved to have a hectic schedule. This was mostly his fault, since he wanted her to try every activity under the sun; dance, theater, girl scouts and every single sport. Eight and a half years after she came around, they decided to make it official.

Married for over two decades, and co-parenting for 30, they had their ups and downs, but were true partners. It wasn't ever easy or seamless, but they both were full of effort, intelligence and accomplishment, as well as so much pure joy. Not a fairytale by any means, but if you asked both of them, they would say it was well worth it.

He was also many things, career-wise, and all of them were purposeful. He was a retiree of the VA, where he was a recreational therapist. Prior to that he did clinical work with other veterans, and civilians, who experienced various forms of PTSD. He was clearly more than qualified from experience, for both of those positions. He took his job very seriously, and modeled what it was like to be dedicated, but also enjoy what he did. The special part of what he did was not in his job description; he became familial to all of his patients, and truly cared about them. He cared so much that he would voluntarily work holidays, because he knew that holidays, while intended to be cheerful occasions, were often the loneliest, if you didn't have family or others to celebrate with. Well-suited for the job, but not a slave to it, he struck a great balance for as long as he served in that role. He missed a few Christmases, Thanksgivings and birthday parties to be there.

Things that I think he would like others to know are just little day-in and day-out tidbits. Flying and traveling always took longer – he had to be 115% prepared, and many flights were missed due to last minute bathroom stops. An accessible home isn't simply just widening the doorways so that a chair can fit. It is also having alternative cabinets, shelving, and so much more to keep things within reach. Of course, not everything fit on lower shelves, so his pride and independence had to be put on the back-burner. He was fully present for all the days of his life and learned there is so much more to life than vanity and superficiality. Functionality and connection trump all.

He went into renal failure at the beginning of 2016, spending over a month in the hospital trying to find the correct diagnosis and then an inpatient rehab facility to regain strength. From then on, he attended dialysis, both in-home and at centers, for over four years and had multiple surgeries to put in ports, shunts, you name it.

In 2018, he was officially diagnosed with Parkinson's Disease. This had been suspected for a while, with tremors and other troubles.

Finally in 2019, a lump was found at the base of his skull and neck, which turned out to be a slow-growing non-Hodgkins lymphoma. He was told he didn't need treatment quite then, and it was just something to keep an eye on.

In April of 2021, after a round-the-clock live-in nurse, several caretakers, and extreme battles with day-to-day living, he succumbed to the combo of health issues that plagued him. Hospice nurses were impressed with the strength and resilience he showed, even in his transition to death. He was surrounded by his three closest ladies; his wife, his sister and his daughter.

He wanted you to know his story, to pave the way for you, whatever your struggles may be. Don't discount your tough times, but don't let them beat you.

He wanted to help whoever he could, however he could, even after he is gone from this world.

He leaves behind a wonderful legacy, and a community that continues to grow and learn from each other.

Rick's grandest wish was for those who find themselves in a similar situation, and wanting to give up, to know and truly understand that there is still so much more out there to explore, do and learn. Life truly does roll on.